THE
NEW
NAKED

THE ULTIMATE
SEX EDUCATION
FOR GROWN-UPS

HARRY FISCH, MD
WITH KAREN MOLINE

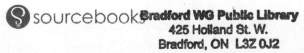 sourcebooks

Bradford WG Public Library
425 Holland St. W.
Bradford, ON L3Z 0J2

Published by Sourcebooks, Inc.
P.O. Box 4410, Naperville, Illinois 60567-4410
(630) 961-3900
Fax: (630) 961-2168
www.sourcebooks.com

Library of Congress Cataloging-in-Publication Data
Fisch, Harry-
  The new naked : ultimate sex education for grown-ups/ Harry Fisch, MD with Karen Moline.
    pages cm
  Includes bibliographical references and index.
(trade : alk. paper) 1. Sex instruction. 2. Sexual disorders. 3. Sex—Psychological aspects. I. Moline, Karen. II. Title.
  HQ31.F6175 2014
  613.9071--dc23

                         2013040165

Printed and bound in the United States of America.
VP 10 9 8 7 6 5 4 3 2 1

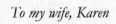

To my wife, Karen

CONTENTS

Introduction: Sex Is a Dipstick   vii

Part I. Sex Talk 101: What's Right and What Can Go Wrong 1

  Lesson 1. Satisfaction: Can You Get It? Yes, You Can!   3

  Lesson 2. What Turns You Off to Sex?   49

  Lesson 3. Erection, Interrupted: The Anatomy of Sexual
    Dysfunction   77

  Lesson 4. Risky Business: Pornography, Affairs, and Sexual
    Addiction   129

Part II. Communication 101: Learning How to Say What
  You Need   167

  Lesson 5. L Is for Listening…So Shut the F**k Up   1/1

  Lesson 6. S Is for Security…So Think about Why You're
    Together   205

  Lesson 7. D Is for Desire…You've Got to Show It to
    Know It   233

Epilogue: Now That You Know What You're Doing…   259

References   261

Index   271

Acknowledgments   283

About the Author   285

INTRODUCTION
SEX IS A DIPSTICK

L et me tell you why I'm writing this book: lots of people are having lots of sex...but that doesn't mean they're having lots of fun doing it.

And I am determined to do something about it.

As one of the most renowned urologists and reproductive specialists in New York City, in practice since 1989, I've seen thousands of patients with sexual dysfunction and sexual satisfaction problems and aching pleas for help. But almost everyone who walked into my office, men and women alike, was more interested in talking about—and being treated for—the one issue that wasn't being talked about anywhere else. They didn't just want to know how to have better sex, but *how to be happy* in their relationships at the same time.

This book will show you that sexual satisfaction and emotional satisfaction are not mutually exclusive in a relationship. That may not sound like rocket science, but you'd be amazed at the number of people who don't think the two are possible to achieve. In fact, you can take simple steps on your own and with your partner to improve all aspects of your life together. This book will show you exactly what to do.

Before we get into that, here's an important note I want to

make as a men's health expert. Women often don't realize that as men get older their sexuality can be affected by many different issues. They're dealing with declining testosterone levels as well as performance issues, weight issues, stress issues, and that old issue of getting older and not getting it up so easily.

These problems have to be acknowledged because they are often the reasons why the sex in these men's relationships goes away or awry. When a woman understands any physiological issues affecting the man in her life, she can be far more effective at helping him make the changes he needs for his health, for his happiness and, most importantly, for the overall health and happiness of their relationship.

How This Book Came to Be

I've already written two books that address the medical aspects of male sexuality and the physical nature of the problems that can occur between partners in a relationship, *The Male Biological Clock: The Startling News about Aging, Sexuality, and Fertility in Men* (published in 2005) and *Size Matters: The Hard Facts about Male Sexuality That Every Woman Should Know* (published in 2008).

What still needs to be talked about candidly, however, is basic sex education for grown-ups. I'm not talking about the mechanics of the sex act itself, but how lack of sexual fulfillment and an inability to even know how to bring up the issue affect a couple's intimacy and togetherness. I've seen this in countless couples that have come into my office. They're talking at each other but not to each other. They're frustrated and upset. They know there's an enormous, sexually charged elephant in the room, but they can't bring it up. They don't have the language to express their needs, and I quickly learned to provide it for them.

What I told these couples is that every relationship has a sex factor and a happiness factor, which are inextricably intertwined. Some people can have a lot of happiness in their relationship without a huge amount of sex. But I have yet to meet a couple that has a happy relationship when the sex is bad, unsatisfying, infrequent, or mechanical.

Sounds ridiculously simple, right? Well, it's not—if you can't talk about it. Back in the Stone Age, when I was in medical school, nobody discussed patients' emotional issues—which is crazy when you think about it today—and nobody *ever* discussed how to be happy. There was little talk about lifestyle and behavior, drugs and drinking, and sexual issues and addiction, all of which have a potent effect on physical health and thus on sexual performance in both men and women.

Yet once I started my practice, suddenly dozens of patients were confiding in me about all of these things. It didn't matter what their medical issues were; the common denominator was their unhappiness about the sexual aspects of their relationship. They sat there, eager and willing, waiting for me to give them a magic bullet to improve their sex life, thinking that Viagra or testosterone or losing weight would do it for them.

But nothing I could prescribe would work if they remained unable to talk about what they really wanted and needed. I quickly realized that prescribing Viagra for mechanical fixes was a mistake if I did not address how to have a great relationship *beyond* the physical aspects.

In fact, I said this just the other day to a pharmaceutical rep who stopped in my office to discuss an order for Viagra. "You know," I told her, "I can't give Viagra to patients anymore without cringing."

I thought for a second that she was going to faint.

"What I mean," I hastened to add, "is that it doesn't seem right to just prescribe Viagra to men having trouble in bed when they don't know what a relationship is about. Viagra might help with the physical part, but if they don't deal with any underlying emotional issues, nothing is going to work."

She regained her composure in a hurry.

In other words, what these men needed was not someone with a quick physical fix for their issues, but someone to help them find and maintain happiness in their sexual relationships. Each man needed the woman in his life—that's *you*, by the way!—to help him see the whole picture.

But here's the catch: these guys, as you doubtless already know, couldn't talk about any of this because they didn't know what to talk about or, more importantly, *how* to. They were like cavemen—they probably knew what they wanted, but they didn't have the language or the ability to make their needs known. Many of them didn't even have simple, basic information about sex and sexual health, and what was normal or not. Plus, there was no one they could ask.

In other words, they were grown men in dire need of *real* sex education.

Not the kind of sex education they may have sniggered through in junior high, with health teachers droning on about zygotes, hormones, and puberty, and all that convoluted medical mumbo jumbo. No, they needed more than just a refresher course in the basics of anatomy. They needed to know that they didn't have to live with sexual unhappiness. They needed someone to tell them how to have good sex and good relationships *for a lifetime*.

That's what *The New Naked* is all about. This is a comprehensive book—written about men but for women—showing how easily you can achieve the sexually satisfying adult relationships you've always wanted.

Nearly all of the books that deal with sexual issues and marriage are psychologically based, written by couples' counselors, psychologists, psychiatrists, or sex therapists. That's great, because there is a real need for those books. None of them, however, gets back to the basics of sex education for adults from a medical perspective like mine as an experienced urologist and fertility and men's health specialist who has also counseled couples for years on their sexual needs and their misperceptions.

Because I've treated infertile couples and male patients for several decades, I've become an expert at candidly dealing with all sorts of sexual and emotional dysfunction. I explore these issues on Howard Stern's Howard 101 channel on SiriusXM, which hosts my radio show every Wednesday night. I also am often consulted as an expert on *The Dr. Oz Show*, where I serve on the medical advisory board. And I've created the websites www.drharryfisch.com and www.harryfisch.com, which discuss male health and sexuality, so the millions of people who need that candid advice can find it easily.

I've written this book for women like you so you can share this information with the man in your life. Once you know what's really wrong, of course, you can start to make it better. But more than just showing you how to spot potential problems, this book talks about what can go right (even if it has already gone wrong) with your emotional relationship and your sex life. It's an essential road map to the best sex and the happiest relationship of your life.

Sex Is the Dipstick of Every Relationship

I always tell my patients that sex is the dipstick of every relationship. That's because sex is wonderful. Sex is fun. Sex is pure pleasure…when it's done right.

In fact, sex is a great indicator of the health of a relationship. Couples who are happy have a regular, mutually satisfying, loving, and uninhibited sex life where they feel utterly at ease in each other's arms. The couples I see usually aren't like that. (Not yet, at least!) And I'm guessing that if you're reading this book, you're interested in making your own sexual relationship work on a more profoundly pleasing level.

Let me tell you a story. Often at dinner parties, someone will ask what I do. As soon as I tell them that I'm a board-certified urologist, specializing in reproductive issues and sexual dysfunction, their eyes light up. They've got questions and an expert sitting right next to them. "So, doc," the man will usually ask, "how often should couples be having sex?"

"Well," I'll start to say. "On average—"

"I had sex two times this month," is usually what I hear when the person confiding in me hastens to interrupt. "And lemme tell ya, it was *fantastic*!"

Now, I'd never burst someone's bubble in public, but having sex twice in a month is on the *very* low side of average. It's not fantastic at all. Something is wrong in that marriage.

"You know," I'll finally say, "sex is the dipstick of any relationship. You have to check it regularly."

"I hear ya! Thanks for the advice!"

My heart sinks, but I don't push it. This husband and wife aren't patients—and obviously, they don't have enough patience to hear my answer. But what I want to tell him is that if you're not having a lot of sex or having bad sex, you have a big problem. It needs to be addressed. It needs to be fixed.

I'll tell you why: as a species, we are biologically programmed to have sex. Not during a specific mating season but *regularly*. Men are genetically hardwired to spread their seed as much as they can in order to ensure the survival of the human race by creating future generations. Biologically speaking, a relationship lacking regular sex is a relationship in danger.

We may have moved on from the time when reproduction was the primary purpose of having sex, but we certainly haven't moved on to a time when sex isn't necessary. It's both a biological imperative to create future generations and an emotional and physical necessity in healthy adults. After all, sex is one of the greatest pleasures in life. Right?

So if you're in a committed relationship and you're *not* having sex, it's *not* normal. Don't assume that's the way it's supposed to be. Lack of sex could mean either partner has medical problems that should be checked out immediately, or perhaps one is having an affair, or in very rare cases, one is gay and not ready to come out of the closet. But most likely, they're not communicating about what they need in bed and what having good sex actually means.

When women tell me they don't want to have sex, I often say that's probably because their sex life hasn't been good. If you've never had good sex—if it's always been a chore or a bore, or it hurts or generally is something that has never given you pleasure—then why would you care about or want to improve your sex drive?

In other words, if you don't want to drive the car, you're not going to fill it up. And you're probably not going to check the dipstick, either. You're more likely to give up on the car and either stop driving or find a different model. That will be the kiss of death for your relationship.

How *The New Naked* Works

There are two parts of *The New Naked*. Think of them as the equivalent of you and your partner going back to school for my version of sex education. It's never too late to learn how to have great sex!

In **Part I. Sex Talk 101: What's Right and What Can Go Wrong**, I'll discuss sexual satisfaction, turn-ons and turn-offs, sexual dysfunction, and sexual risks. This is the information you need, the kind of accurate information that's hard to get.

- **Lesson 1. Satisfaction: Can You Get It? Yes, You Can!** tackles the issue of doing sex right from an emotional point of view. I'll discuss masturbation and how it affects sexual performance, how important lubrication is, and the reasons behind performance anxiety.
- **Lesson 2. What Turns You Off to Sex?** deals with the many ways that couples can lose their spark and get turned off instead of turned on.
- **Lesson 3. Erection, Interrupted: The Anatomy of Sexual Dysfunction** covers the physiological aspects of sexual

dysfunction: how a penis works, what can go wrong, testosterone issues, infertility, and sexually transmitted infections.

- **Lesson 4. Risky Business: Pornography, Affairs, and Sexual Addiction** gets to the heart of a key risk factor that causes a lot of sexual unhappiness—the over-reliance on porn in the twentieth century and what it's doing to real relationships. I'll also discuss how affairs and sexual addiction can destroy relationships.

In **Part II. Communication 101: Learning How to Say What You Need**, I'll introduce my LSD system. It is written for women, but your partner should read some sections on his own or with you.

LSD isn't about the drug, obviously—it stands for Listening + Security + Desire. Mastering these three elements will instantly improve your and your partner's ability to communicate with each other. Finally, both of you will be able to talk freely, openly, and honestly about what you really want and what you really need. Once you can do that, you'll be able to get more sex. Better sex. Mutually satisfying sex.

But unless you and your partner are willing to delve into what makes your relationship tick, you'll never have a satisfying sex life. Even if you are the most skilled lover in the world, your relationship will falter if it's based only on sexual attraction. I firmly believe that the whole point of your emotional life as an adult is to have an intimate and trusting relationship with somebody who cares about you.

Caring will always be at the core. You can have crazy, hot, passionate sex, but if you don't have the intimacy brought about by mutual love and caring for each other's well-being, the relationship is not going to last. And if you can't identify what it takes to make you happy, your partner sure won't be able to. How do you expect that relationship to work?

This explains why the first element of LSD is Listening. As a woman, you're probably skilled at listening, but being a good listener is actually extremely difficult for men. Most likely, you already know that your guy is not exactly a champion at listening to you, right? In addition to that, guys often forget to acknowledge a woman's need for security, which is as much an innate necessity for most women as the need to "mate" and spread their seed is for most men. Finally, it's incredibly hard for many men to understand and fulfill a woman's desires and to know how to masterfully create and play out sexual fantasies or cravings that will enhance, not destroy, their relationships.

- **Lesson 5. L Is for Listening** will teach your man how to listen—and yes, it's a skill. Men may balk at learning it because they know, deep down, that they stink at it. (They're so used to *not* listening, in fact, that sometimes they are masters at closing off their ears!) This lesson will also teach him when he should keep quiet, when he can and should speak up, and how he can decode the messages you are sending to eliminate misunderstandings.

- **Lesson 6. S Is for Security** talks about the issue that breaks up more marriages than practically anything else: money. Whether we like it or not, money makes the world go around. But it is amazing to me how my patients don't talk candidly to each other about finances and the need for financial and emotional security—and then they can't understand why they're always fighting about money-related issues. We'll tackle that here so you and your partner don't take it out on each other in the bedroom.

- **Lesson 7. D Is for Desire** shows your man how to make you feel special, loved, appreciated, and desired—and *why it's worth his while* to do so. He will learn that a small amount of well-placed, well-timed, and well-meaning effort can reap surprisingly enormous rewards! And you will learn the surprising ways in which this can enhance your sex life, too.

One of the reasons I created the LSD system is that it allows me to cut to the chase when talking to patients. I once got a terrific compliment from a patient's wife who told me I saved her marriage. She said that she got more helpful information from me in just a few appointments than she had in all the years she'd gone to therapy. The reason for her kind words is simple: I only have about thirty minutes with each patient.

I don't have the luxury of time to delve into the whys and who did whats. I need to get to the aha moments in a flash, or my patients won't get the help they need. And I can tell from their faces that with this method, they get it. They go home and they work on what I've instructed them to do. And then they report back to me on their success. That success is a vastly improved relationship—and sex life.

I've taken the best and most useful of all these moments and put them into this book, because it's my mission to get everyone juiced up again. When couples come to see me, I always give them more information about their sexual behavior than they thought they needed when they first came in the door. That's because I know they need it.

In fact, they're amazed at what I tell them, even about the simplest things. Like what to cut out of their diet to lose weight and have more stamina in bed. Like how to put the vibrator away. Like what a woman really wants—which often is as simple as sex with someone who shows, with just a little effort, that he cares about her.

At the very least, both men and women want LSD as the foundation for the best sex and the best relationship they can possibly have. (Even if the men complain that listening is harder than they thought because they never had to do it before!)

I hear the same thing every time I sit before the microphone on my radio show. Callers from all over the country confide their sexual secrets to me anonymously. You know what I hear over and over again? The same questions as from my patients. What's normal for sex? Why can't I satisfy my partner? What am I doing wrong? How do I do this? We don't talk anymore; why won't she talk to me? Am I addicted to porn? Why can't I last as long as I used to? Why am I lasting *too* long? I gained weight, so is that why my sex life stinks? Where can I go for information? Can you help me?

Yes, I can!

Read on, and allow me to help you, too.

PART I

SEX TALK 101

What's Right and What Can Go Wrong

LESSON 1

SATISFACTION
CAN YOU GET IT? YES, YOU CAN!

I f you can't get no satisfaction, you are either having bad sex or not enough sex.

It's that simple.

Here's an example from one of my patients. Walt came into my office, sat down, and sighed. I soon found out why. He was having sex once every four months with his wife. (That's pretty much saying he wasn't having any sex with her.) We went over why this was going on, and Walt's problem turned out to be premature ejaculation, a very common problem for men of all ages. I'll get to that later in this lesson, but essentially premature ejaculation means that a man ejaculates way too quickly. When that happens, the sex act itself can be awfully short and awfully unsatisfying for the woman. Let me just say that his wife Sally was not happy about the current state of their sex life.

What was the reason for Walt's situation? I didn't know yet, but what typically happens is that the guy tells me everything is fine and he lasts a long time, while his partner looks dumbfounded and then says, "Actually, he finishes kind of quickly." When I tell them that typically having sex takes about five to ten minutes and that men with premature ejaculation are done within two minutes, the facial expressions change. He'll look crestfallen and she'll be relieved—that there's a name for his problem and that it's not her fault. And that someone believes her!

Walt's answer was more like denial. He didn't believe he had a problem in the sack. Rather, he thought the problem was on his wife's end. "Talk to my wife," Walt told me. "I really want to have more sex with her."

"I don't think she wants to have sex with *you*," I replied. "Not the way you're doing it now. Everybody wants to have sex. They want things that are pleasurable. So when a woman says that she doesn't want to have sex, it's because it's not pleasurable to her."

Walt looked stunned. And then sheepish.

Fortunately, Sally was eager to talk to me and actually relieved that Walt's problem was such a common one. Together, we were able to pinpoint the causes of Walt's ejaculation problem and get their sex life back on track. Walt just needed a bit of guidance to realize that his sexual issue *wasn't* normal, and that although it was fine for him, it absolutely wasn't fine for his wife. He couldn't last long enough to satisfy Sally, and he was lousy in bed. The problem was that Sally didn't know how to broach the topic without hurting his feelings. When we finally cleared the air, I was able to guide them through the problem and they were able to solve it together.

Yes, Sex Is a Skill, and Yes, You Can Get Better at It

No one wants to think that he or she might be terrible in bed. But many people are because no one ever taught them the basics of good sex. You might be technically proficient. But that doesn't mean the satisfaction level is there. And it's time to do something about it.

Like Sally, the wives who talk to me are desperate to unburden their worries about their sex lives to somebody who understands what's going on in their bedrooms. They've literally been going crazy because they know they need help—because their husbands really need help—and they don't know where to turn. These women aren't embarrassed or ashamed. They're *thrilled* because they have a lethal secret.

The lethal secret is that for them, the sex stinks.

When I tell them the key to unlocking this secret is to treat the physical act of sex as a skill to be learned and to treat their emotions with the LSD you'll learn about in Part II, I see the tension drain out of them, replaced by a hopeful smile. As I mentioned in the Introduction, my patients usually come to me for a quick fix to their flagging sex lives and end up getting a lot more—the information that will help them the most. Most likely, they think a prescription for Viagra or testosterone will solve things, yet they have no clue whether they actually *need* Viagra.

I tell patients like this that sex is like learning how to ski. Even if you're a world-class athlete, you've got to start at the beginning and go down the bunny slope. Basics first. One step at a time. If you think you know what you're doing and blithely hop on the lift to the black-diamond run before you're ready, it can kill you or at least make you look very foolish.

Unsatisfying sex isn't going to kill you physically, but it sure can kill your relationship. A really sad fact is that up to 50 percent of women don't have orgasms during sex. Another sad fact is that about 45 percent of men have premature ejaculations.

Putting the two together is a recipe for no fun in bed for either of you.

Yet everyone seems to think that simply because you *can* have sex, you will automatically have *great* sex. I've seen so much sadness and frustration from people who love each other but can't please each other in bed that it's become my responsibility to teach my patients how to have good sex, because it's instantly clear that *they don't know how to do it.* They simply don't understand that while good sex is a skill, great sex takes even more mastery. And having a thriving, loving relationship with great sex whenever you want it is a lifetime endeavor. One, I can happily say from experience, that is an awful lot of fun to master!

Take Bobby, for example. He sat in my office with a mopey expression.

"I don't know what I'm doing wrong," he confessed. "Most of my girlfriends tell me they don't have orgasms during sex, but they won't tell me what they want me to do. I feel like a complete failure."

"This is actually a very common problem," I told him. "Did you know that 50 percent of women can't achieve orgasm through vaginal penetration? So there's no reason to think you're alone with this issue. Everyone thinks there's a mechanical aspect to good sex, but with women, that's just not how things work.

"Here's the good news," I went on. "The solution is actually simpler than you think. Next time you're having sex, ask your girlfriend what she wants and which position she prefers. Tell her you want to make her happy, and you'd love for her to show you. It is very common for women to only be able to come to orgasm in one specific position, but believe it or not, sometimes they're too shy or inhibited or embarrassed to say so. Help them communicate better, and your own performance will get better, too."

That means, don't be shy. If you want something, speak up. It can be hard in the throes of lovemaking to say or do everything you want, so if the opportunity passes you by, bring it up afterward when you're both feeling relaxed, and be sure to remind your partner about it before the next time you have sex.

Is This You?
If You Don't Speak Up, Your Partner Will Never Know

Suzanne and John sat in my office with long faces.

"I was able to have an orgasm with my other boyfriend, but not with John," Suzanne said.

"Okay, so what position did you prefer with your prior boyfriend?" I asked.

"Oh, it was me on top so there was deeper penetration," she explained.

"Have you tried that with John?" I asked, even though I already knew the answer.

"Um, no."

"Why not?" I asked, even though I already knew that answer, too.

"Well, I didn't want to bring it up."

What was she waiting for? If you don't bring it up, how can you expect your partner to automatically know what to do? Communicate. It's really that simple. Suzanne didn't have to tell John, "Well, I did it like this with my other boyfriend, and it made me come every time." That might hurt John's feelings and make him feel that he was being compared to another lover (never a good concept, obviously). All she had to do is point him in the right direction by saying, "Let's try this." John also could have asked what she would like him to do. That might have helped her to tell him candidly without the ex-boyfriend comparison.

The Number One Question I'm Asked: How Often Is Normal?

The average man has eleven erections every day (including partial erections). Teenage boys and men in their twenties with high hormonal levels may think that having sex several times a day is totally normal. Otherwise, the typical average is two to three times a week. That was also the figure from the American Sexual Behavior Study, a 2006 survey reporting that the average frequency of sex for married couples went from about once every two to three days for couples between the ages of eighteen and twenty-nine, to about twice a week for couples between thirty and fifty, and less than once a week for older couples.

In the early phase of a love relationship, couples of any age tend to have a lot of sex—daily, if not more frequently. But the frequency of sex declines as any relationship ages, although married couples have more sex than those who are single. Obviously, regular access to sex makes it more likely to happen!

Remember, these are averages. Some couples are happy with more frequent sex, while some are happy with less frequent sex.

If you only feel like having sex once or twice a week but find those encounters deeply satisfying, that's normal for *you* and that's totally fine. Not wanting *any* sex is not.

And that's really the point: not how much sex you're having, but whether you and your partner are happy with the sex you *are* having. Quality wins out over quantity every time. It's all about the satisfaction.

That said, quality sex isn't just about frequency. It's also about the length of the sex act.

There have been studies in which couples consented to be scientifically observed having sex while an observer timed each session with a stopwatch to make a fairly accurate assessment about the length of the coupling. Not surprisingly, the time it takes a couple to have sex varies widely, ranging from the excessively short (about two minutes or less, which famed sex researcher Alfred Kinsey dryly noted was a "frequent source of marital conflict") to the "Are you done yet?" (over forty minutes).

An astonishing 45 percent of men finish the sex act too quickly, which is to say, within two minutes. That's quite speedy. *Way* too speedy for the average woman to be able to have an orgasm through vaginal penetration alone. At least five minutes, and more like seven, is usually what's needed for a woman to be able to achieve orgasm.

And even though the average length of the average inter-vaginal sex session is about 7.3 minutes, that's still not particularly long, especially for women, who usually take much longer than men to become aroused enough to have an orgasm.

So whether your man is done within two minutes of things getting hot and heavy or still not done forty minutes later, you may want to gently broach the idea of getting a medical checkup to make sure everything's functioning correctly. And don't worry, if 7.3 minutes doesn't seem like enough time for you to get the satisfaction you need, Part II of this book will teach you and your partner better communication skills so you both can be happy in bed and out.

How Often Do Couples Have Sex?

So how often do couples really have sex? In case you're interested, the American Sexual Behavior Study of 2006 found these numbers about sexual frequency:

Married Couples	
Age	**Frequency of Sex (average number of times yearly)**
18-29	109.1
30-39	87.0
40-49	70.2
50-59	52.5
60-69	32.2
70+	17.2
Unmarried Couples	
Age	**Frequency of Sex (average number of times yearly)**
18-29	73.4
30-39	67.8
40-49	48.2

50-59	29.3
60-69	16.2
70+	3.3

When Was the Last Time You Were Taught Anything about Sex?

Most people start learning about sex and reproduction in middle school, right when puberty hits, hormones are flying, and bodies are changing. But no one actually talks about the act of sex or how to do it safely and do it well. When I was growing up, we snuck copies of *Playboy*, thinking this would teach us all we needed to know.

Nowadays, with easy access to the online world of porn and YouTube videos, kids are "learning" about sex—and seeing it in far more graphic ways than I could have imagined at their age— long before they're emotionally ready. Not only that, but the distorted, fake, fantastical sex exhibited in porn can have a huge detrimental effect on young men watching it, who begin to expect their own partners to look and behave like porn stars. (I'll discuss this in detail in Lesson 4.)

However, most schools haven't changed how they talk about sex, except to add information about HIV and other sexually transmitted diseases. Teachers go through the basics of biology and anatomy, and as teens get older, perhaps they are taught the mechanics of reproduction, how the sperm meets the egg, and so on, often along with stern admonitions about abstinence (something teens with raging hormones are unlikely to process). But none of this teaches people how to have sex in a safe, healthy, and rewarding way.

The vast majority of us are going to have sex at some point in our lives. Most likely, that will start in our late teenage years or as young adults. So who teaches teens and young adults how to have sex? Who can you ask? If you think about it, there are very few trustworthy or well-informed sources for most people.

As a result, we turn to friends, older siblings, and the media, along with the newest source of endlessly streaming information—the Internet. All of these sources may mean well, but they usually are completely wrong about how to do things. Sure, if they're uninhibited about it, friends and siblings can talk about what works for them, but that doesn't mean their advice will be good for you. And they may not be telling you the entire truth because they're too embarrassed to admit that they don't exactly know what they're doing!

In addition, the sexual images plastered all over the media of porn stars and Hollywood stars with impossibly perfect bodies offer such a fake, idealized version of sex and how real bodies look and behave that young people are often more embarrassed and inhibited by these "lessons" than empowered to approach sex with partners in healthy ways. Young people simply believe that they'll never measure up to those fantasy standards.

Put simply, the Internet is a hotbed of well-intentioned but often seriously wrong "facts" about sex and how to do it. The danger is that many people believe what they read on the Internet about sex is far more accurate than it actually is. Does this mean you should never go online for advice? Of course not. But it does mean that you should only get advice from reputable, medically sound sources like my websites and those of other sexual health experts, as well as the federal Centers for Disease Control and Prevention, or the Mayo Clinic.

Proof of this lack of knowledge came when I did a salon at *Cosmopolitan* magazine in 2008 called "Sex Education for Adults." The questions I received from the smart, educated, sexually experienced women in the audience floored me. Why does semen taste sweet? How often should I be having sex? Can I masturbate too much? Is it harming our relationship? Don't men always orgasm before women do? How can you tell if a guy is good in bed? And many more. Many of these questions were really basic, but I'd say that 90 percent of the people in the room couldn't answer any of them. And if they couldn't, there was little hope for the rest of us.

As you know, I'm writing this book because I want to rectify this lack of knowledge. So for everyone looking for answers to these types of questions and more, read on.

Great Foreplay Doesn't Start in the Bedroom— It Starts First Thing in the Morning

How does great sex start?

With foreplay.

When does foreplay start?

The minute you wake up in the morning.

It also starts when your partner puts the dishes in the dishwasher. Really. I can't tell you how many female radio callers say they'd probably have an orgasm in the kitchen if their husbands put away the silverware!

Yes, something as mundane as participating in those boring daily chores is foreplay. This kind of foreplay shows that your partner cares about sharing the workload around the house (and vice versa). It demonstrates that you are equals, instead of you being expected to take care of the kids and the house and go to work and then listen to your man moan about his boss and how hard his day was.

In other words, the more he helps make your household run smoothly, the more you are going to love him for it. That's a nice way to set the mood, isn't it? After all, who'd want to have sex with someone who can't be bothered to clean up his mess? Or, on occasion, *your* mess?

I'll discuss this concept in much greater detail in Part II, but suffice it to say that the best kind of foreplay starts when you both wake up and continues throughout the day. For example, a man should call his partner when she least expects it. To say that he's thinking of you. Or if it's not a good time to interrupt, he can send surreptitious, loving, teasing texts. Minimal effort—honestly, how long does it take to send a text?—can reap enormous rewards. A woman who is thinking about her partner's thoughtfulness will be loving and happy to see him when he walks in the door that night.

Because where does foreplay really take place? For women especially, foreplay starts in your brain. It isn't physical. In fact, it's everything but, leading up to you or your partner creating so much desire that good sex is the welcome result. Here's an example: A man shows you that he cares by being kind and thoughtful. He acknowledges your needs and desires during the day. He knows how important it is to be present, which means not checking his email when he's on the phone with you. He compliments your shoes even if he's seen them a hundred times, or your hair even if it's a bit of a mess. He doesn't interrupt your discussions to take a call.

He shows you he cares by simply saying I love you in little ways like this—and *meaning it*. (Let's not underestimate the need for these efforts to be genuine. Women can tell when they are being patronized or being given "lip service.") So by the time you get to the bedroom, you're already in the mood.

Foreplay isn't just about sex—it's about *life*. And in Part II, I'll show you how to get your partner to listen better, to make you feel more secure and to increase your desire—the LSD—so you'll be able to state your needs clearly and easily. He'll hear what you're saying. He'll want to make you feel secure and loved…and yes, you'll both be flooded with desire.

I see this all the time in the medical world. You can be the smartest neurosurgeon on the planet, but if your bedside manner stinks and you make it clear that you're too important or too busy for your patients, you're a failure as a doctor. Your patients will see that you don't genuinely care about them, and they won't trust you or feel comfortable being treated by you. This can lead to serious complications for them—and for you as the doctor trying to do your job and help them. I learned the importance of this concept when I ran the medical-school urology course at Columbia University College of Physicians and Surgeons from 2002 to 2007 and was told to teach "humanism" as part of the curriculum.

I had no idea what humanism was and I didn't know who to ask, so I decided to put the question to my smarty-pants medical students. Oops. They didn't know, either. Nobody explained it. So over the five years of teaching, I had students write essays on what they thought humanism meant in medicine. After about two years, I began to understand. Humanism is nothing more than showing how much you care about others.

The same thing applies to sex. Men need to learn humanism toward their partners—namely, *you*! And also to realize that sex isn't just about their needs and their erection. Once you both start practicing more humanism in your relationship, it will transfer directly into your sex life.

Practice—and Practice Well

Great sex isn't just about mastering foreplay. One of the easiest ways to become a more accomplished lover is to have more sex. But here's the catch. It has to be *good* sex.

I was on a football team in high school that didn't win any games. We were about the worst team ever. But one thing that Coach said all the time resonated in a huge way, not just about football but about everything in life. "Practice doesn't make perfect," he told us. "*Perfect* practice makes perfect."

If you keep practicing anything badly, especially sex, you're not going to like it and neither will your partner. Sex will become a chore. I often hear women say, "I don't want to have sex. I'm too tired." That means they're not having good sex. Because if your whole day is a miserable drudge, but you know you're going to have good sex later, you look forward to it, regardless of how tired you are.

Look at it this way: I play a lot of tennis. I practice and take lots of lessons. They're important lessons; I'm thinking about every shot and I work to make each one the best possible. But the real reason to keep practicing is that once I'm in the game, I *don't* want to be thinking too much or I'll miss every ball. I have to relax, trust that I learned the lessons well, and hope that muscle memory will take over.

It is the same with sex. You should "practice" and explore and try different things with your partner. But if you're thinking too much about the mechanics of what you're doing during your actual lovemaking sessions, you're not going to relax and enjoy what's happening at that moment.

This is why it's so important to know your body, know your preferences, know your partner's preferences, and most of all, to speak up about what feels good.

If you have a hard time saying what you want, do a sex checklist. List what you want from your partner, such as "I want a massage," "I want a dim room," "Being on top is my favorite position," or "This is my fantasy: (and spell it out)." Then ask him to do the same.

I've found that women tend to want their partners to concentrate more on foreplay, while men often just want to get going. Have some fun figuring out how to make each other happy by practicing the items on your checklist. Alternate your wishes with his, and then go back to the beginning and repeat. After a while, you'll both be getting exactly what you want. Then write out a new checklist!

Masturbation = ~~Satisfaction~~ Frustration

Since I've just discussed humanism and caring and, yes, his erections, let's move to a topic that's all about his penis, his hands, and why he's placing them on himself when he should be placing them on you. Namely, masturbation.

Not so many eons ago, when humans were rutting in jungles and caves, their top priority wasn't silk sheets or mood music or whether the door was locked to keep the kids out, but surviving through another threat-filled day. Sex had to be quick and productive because there wasn't a lot of time to make love when you knew that a woolly mammoth or saber-toothed tiger might be stalking you any minute, ready to pounce.

Nowadays, we don't have to rush sex unless we deliberately sneak out for a quickie on our lunch hour. Instead, we can concentrate on pleasuring each other. But orgasms can be elusive for couples when ejaculation problems caused by masturbation ruin the mood.

A predictable saga unfolded when a patient named Sam came to see me. He was forty-four, overweight, and wanted to feel better. He assumed that he had low testosterone levels, and he was right. But he thought that a prescription for testosterone would be an instant, automatic fountain of youth. I didn't tell him right away that hormone therapy wouldn't benefit him that much. After all, he was asking for help, and the first step was to get his male hormones stabilized. Once they were at normal levels, I could tell him about the satisfaction stuff.

Once the blood work was back, we discussed Sam's numbers and the improvements I'd seen. The testosterone had kicked in quickly, and he had more energy and more sex drive. Then I told him bluntly that both would be even better if he lost weight.

"No bread, pizza, pasta, cookies, and cakes. No salt and sugar," I told him.

"Come on," he said, "that's all I wanna eat."

"Well, that's what you've got to work on," I replied. "Start slow. Cut out one bagel a day. It's nothing but junk flour and salt. You don't need it."

"Bagels have salt?" he said.

"Yes, a lot. Bread is full of salt. Fat's not the enemy—sugar is.

And too much salt. Always taste your food before you sprinkle salt on it."

I could see him mulling this over, so I moved to the next point and asked, "Now that you're feeling better, what about your sex life? How often are you having sex with your wife?"

"Every couple of months or so," he said quickly.

Which meant *never*

"Okay," I said, "why do you think that is?"

"I don't know, doc. Maybe you could talk to my wife."

"I'd be happy to, but let me just say that no woman is going to want to have sex that isn't pleasurable. Are you using enough lubrication?"

"Sure, she's lubricated, everything like that."

"So what do you think is the problem?"

"Well, I kinda last a long time. When we do have sex, she has an orgasm or whatever," Sam added. I wasn't sure if he was telling the truth or not. "Then she turns around and waits for me to finish."

Aha, here we go. "How often do you masturbate?" I asked. "Once a day, once every two days? Are you good at it?"

He smiled smugly. "I'm *very* good at it."

There it was—the reason why they never had sex. If a man tells me he's a great lover because he lasts forever, I know there's a satisfaction problem for his partner. She may have had an orgasm, be feeling great, and just want the sex to end and to have a lovely long hug before bed. But he'll still be going at it.

If he's been watching too much porn (which I'll get to in Lesson 4), he may be thinking that's the only way to be "great" in bed. Most porn movies feature extensive scenes where the men pump and pump and pump and the women moan in "ecstasy."

In truth, they're all faking it and likely thinking of nothing more satisfying than hearing the director say, "Cut."

Or, like Sam, he could be equating great sex with how frequently he can ejaculate, because he was used to copious ejaculations through masturbation. Which is another *very* common mistake. But as we'll see in the next section, since his masturbation was all about this ejaculation, he couldn't ejaculate when he was with his wife any more.

Needless to say, Sam had a lot of work to do on his sexual skills. Sure, he was brilliant at pleasuring himself—to the detriment of pleasuring his wife. His technique was fine for a horny fifteen-year-old but not for an adult who wanted a satisfying relationship and sex life. He needed a refresher course on how to have good mutual sex, pronto!

Hands On: Men and Masturbation

Let's take a step back and look at the psychology and physiology behind masturbating. Masturbation, or self-pleasuring, is as normal a human activity as walking or talking. Infant boys typically discover that fondling their penis feels good, and infant girls discover the marvels of their vaginas. They may play with themselves often unless prevented from doing so by adults. (Of course they don't ejaculate until puberty and the maturation of the genitals.) In short, masturbation is a healthy, pleasurable activity that men and women of all ages engage in, whether they're in an active relationship or not.

I've found that women don't like to talk about their partner's masturbation habits and usually underestimate how much of it goes on regularly. Some men engage in it a lot. I'm not talking about teenage boys whose intense hormonal surges make masturbation practically a necessary relief during puberty. I'm talking about normal, sexually fulfilled men. Not surprisingly, younger men tend to masturbate more often than older men. Men who don't have a regular partner masturbate more often, too, again not surprisingly.

In other words, masturbation is totally normal. A recent study by the Kinsey Institute found that nearly 85 percent of men living with a sexual partner reported masturbating in the past year. The same study found that 45 percent of women in a relationship masturbate. After the first erotic phase of a relationship subsides, people discover that they aren't always horny at the same time.

Masturbation can fill the need for sexual release. Feel free to go at it if you're traveling on your own and you miss your partner and you're horny. It's certainly better than picking up someone in a bar. Masturbation is especially encouraged for women who have had trouble with orgasms in the past and need to become better acquainted with their body so they know what it takes to please themselves. (They can then share this delightful information with their partners.)

But—and this is one of the *biggest* buts in the whole book—masturbation can become an enormous problem in your relationship if one partner gets so used to self-pleasuring that he or she can't get aroused by regular sex any more. If that happens to your sex life or your partner's sex life, it's time to take action.

That's because there's a potential psychological hazard

to masturbation. Sex, as you know, is about a whole lot more than just the physical aspect of orgasm. What's so wonderful about sex is how it engages all of your five senses: sight, by how you see your partner; hearing, by the murmurs and whispers and pleasurable sighs you both are (or at least *should)* be making; taste, by the deliciousness of kissing each other's body parts; smell, by all the evocative scents emanating from your bodies; and touch, by how you feel and explore and caress and hug. Each of these stimuli helps to make sex an incredibly pleasurable experience.

What happens when people masturbate, however, is that they concentrate specifically on the orgasm part, not the rest of it. Sense of touch is obviously highly engaged, and personal noises and fantasies are running through the mind, but the masturbator is only enjoying these senses on his or her own. They're unique to the masturbation experience and can't be shared.

Masturbation can only be a solitary pursuit. It's fine on occasion but shouldn't be a regular part of your sexual repertoire, especially if it begins to interfere with your sexual activities with your partner. In other words, chronic masturbation isn't great if you or your partner is using it as your primary source of sexual pleasure. A chronic masturbator knows what gets things going quickly—like props or sex toys or certain locations—and can stimulate in exactly that way. Usually, this means a pretty zippy ride between initial thought and ejaculation. Great for him when he's in the mood for a "wank," as they say in Britain about quick climaxes. Not good for you when you're in the mood for a lovely, long lovemaking session.

Here's the kicker: A penis that has grown accustomed to a particular kind of sensation leading to rapid ejaculation will not work the same way when it's aroused differently. Orgasm is delayed or doesn't happen at all, often leaving you both frustrated and sometimes even feeling like failures. Women may blame themselves, thinking perhaps they're not desirable or skilled at lovemaking. Men may think there's something wrong with their performance. The truth is, the more your partner relies on his solo skills, the more his couple skills skid to a halt.

This happens to many more couples than you would think. Once you and your partner master the listening skills in Part II, you'll be better able to state your needs, and he will be better able to hear and act on them.

Too Little: Premature Ejaculation

On the opposite end of the time-to-orgasm spectrum was Edward, who came to me saying he wanted Viagra. After I determined that he was perfectly healthy and had no erectile dysfunction, I asked him about his sex life. He said that he rarely had sex with his wife and went to prostitutes instead. Wondering how this related to his desire for Viagra, I asked how long he lasted during sex. His answer was, "Less than a minute." In other words, he had premature ejaculation.

As we discussed it further, the pieces started to come together. He *wanted* to have sex with his wife, but he worried that his premature ejaculation would upset her. That wasn't a problem with the prostitutes, who pretended all was well and gushed over his manliness. Of course, a prostitute or a mistress won't tell a client that his blink-and-you-miss-it pumping isn't satisfying. She's getting compensated not to.

Edward had no idea he could be treated so that he could last longer in bed, please his wife, and stop seeing strangers for sex. If he wanted to save his marriage, he needed to understand that sex was about his relationship with his wife and not about a quick orgasm with a paid stranger.

He also had no idea the average man lasted about seven times longer than he did. At the time, I don't think he cared to know because he was deep in denial. He thought he was a stud.

But if a man can't satisfy his partner and can *only* satisfy himself by going to prostitutes or masturbating, how do you think his partner feels? Awfully upset, of course. Not only are they unsatisfied, but their lover is going elsewhere for satisfaction. Yet women in this position often feel responsible for not pleasing their lover…that something's wrong with *them*. Not surprisingly, this can lead to friction, frustration, and fighting, which further reduces both partners' chances for good sex.

I realized this was probably the case with Edward and his wife when I asked, "Can you bring your wife with you next time?"

"Huh?" he said. "Are you kidding me?" He clearly wasn't thinking about her needs.

I explained that it was extremely important for me to also treat his partner, adding that nearly every case of premature ejaculation has a simple explanation. It's one of the most common types of male sexual dysfunction, affecting 20 to 30 percent of all men. In fact, premature ejaculation is a reflex, *not* a psychological abnormality.

Dear Dr. Fisch: Is Chronic Masturbation Cheating?

Dear Dr. Fisch,

I know my husband thinks about other women when he's jerking off. This is driving me crazy because it feels to me like he's cheating. Am I wrong to get so steamed?

Signed, Hands Off

Dear Hands Off,

Some women I've spoken to think of masturbating as cheating. You may wonder why, but the answer is easy. They know that their partners are indulging in whatever flights of fancy are needed to help them get their rocks off. This might mean fantasies about their second-grade teacher, the hot neighbor next door when they were teenagers, the red-haired executive assistant at work who is happily married and the mother of three, the yoga teacher with the most flexible spine in the Western hemisphere, the sultry actress with the perfect figure you'll never have, the porn star with the surgically enhanced body you'll never have (and never would have even if you could afford it!)… You get where I'm going with this.

My advice is: Don't look for other problems when you don't have them. Instead, take a step back and assess the real problem. I understand your frustration with your husband, and I wonder if you're looking for something to blame him for doing. Chronic

masturbation may be a very real problem in your relationship, but it's a fantasy issue, not a *cheating* problem.

The important questions to ask are: Why do you
think this is such a problem? Does your husband name
the objects of his fantasies when he's masturbating?
Does he ask you to watch and then not want to have
sex with you? Is he doing it in places that might not be
appropriate? Or is he possibly masturbating to avoid
having sex with *you*?

If so, you need to deal with those realities, but you
also have to take the fantasy aspect of masturbation in stride. Fantasy is an integral component of all
sexual relationships, as pretend scenarios can stave
off bedroom boredom—within reason, of course. It's
unrealistic to expect your partner to never fantasize,
but it's also unrealistic and unfair to you if you know
his mind is straying every time you're in bed together.

If, after you've tried this, your partner's fantasizing
continues to bother you, perhaps you could ask him
to fantasize about *you* instead. The last thing you
want him to say is, "I'm not going to have sex if I can't
fantasize the way I want to!" And that way, you know
he's thinking about you and you only.

Technically speaking, premature ejaculation is when a man
loses control over his ejaculation before or just after sexual penetration, often with minimal sexual stimulation. It used to be
defined as being unable to have sex for more than two minutes
without ejaculating, but this figure is being revised downward to

one minute. Premature ejaculation often happens with minimal sexual stimulation.

There are different ways to control this problem:

- By masturbating a *lot* less. A man will in essence un train his penis from ejaculating quickly through self-stimulation.
- By switching sex positions, using extra lubrication to lessen the friction, or trying the stop-and-start technique while having sex.
- By using medication or a product to lessen sensitivity. The effectiveness of these medications provides further proof that premature ejaculation is a central brain and nervous system issue that can be fixed.
- By taking an extremely low dose of an antidepressant medication such as Zoloft. There's virtually no antidepressant effect at such a low dose. The typical dose for clinical depression is 200 milligrams per day, while for premature ejaculation, it's only 25 to 50 milligrams. I don't know who discovered this fortunate side effect, but he or she is to be thanked by all the men it's helped!

Still, lots of men don't want to go to a doctor like me to ask for help and get a prescription. They'd rather go to the drugstore and pick something up over the counter (OTC, or non-prescription). This is not a smart move because self-diagnosis can be nothing more than a waste of money. (Expensive, ineffective vitamins or energy supplements that are merely excreted in urine make for very pricey pee!) In the worst-case scenario, these OTC remedies can have severe, even life-threatening results. For example, an

OTC drug could interfere with medications you're already taking or may be harmful itself if taken in improper doses.

Hands On: Women and Masturbation

In my years of medical practice, 95 percent of the men I've seen or treated masturbate, and many of them have no problem admitting it. But women, as I've said, are much less willing to talk about self-pleasuring—their own or their partner's. Even in the twenty-first century, many women have told me that they were taught that their bodies were "dirty" or that "nice girls don't touch themselves down there," leading to lots of guilt and shame. Plus, if you haven't been taught about anatomy—the function of the clitoris, the difference between vaginal and clitoral orgasms, and so on—you may be less inclined to explore the wonders of your nether regions when the mood strikes.

Another reason some women neglect self-pleasuring is that they think of their system "down there" as annoying because their monthly periods are messy or downright painful, or both. If you have cramps that make you bloated and tender or you experience mood swings related to your period for one week every month, you're probably not going to be in the mood for some hands-on fun "down there."

How women feel about their bodies and their openness to freely discussing anatomy, sexual desire, and self-pleasuring are in large part shaped by the media. Watch any TV show on a network that targets women (especially college-age women), and you'll see an endless repetition of commercials touting tampons and pads and antidepressants and alcohol and feminine hygiene products (which should be pulled from the market, in my opinion, because they can easily cause irritation and make women feel that their natural body odors, or lack thereof, need to be covered up with a chemical spray).

The message is clear: a woman's body has "odors" that should be masked. A woman has "medical conditions" that need drugs so she can get better. A woman can "have fun" only if she's drinking some trendy kind of alcohol. Honestly, if an alien came to earth and saw only those commercials, he'd think that the women of our planet have serious issues with their bodies and their health! It really is a shame that so many women internalize these advertiser-driven messages that their bodily functions are off-kilter or embarrassing, and that their natural scent is something that needs to be washed away. If you come to believe that your vagina is something that's sort of gross, then why would you want to touch it?

I believe that every woman should be able to bring herself to orgasm. This is an extremely important aspect of having a happy and healthy sexual relationship. You need to know which positions and techniques are most pleasurable for your needs, and you need to be able to share these needs with your partner so he knows what to do to satisfy you. Some women can orgasm incredibly quickly, and some women take longer. If you don't know your own anatomy, if you don't know what to expect, and if you don't practice at it, how will you ever know what will bring you the most joy in bed? It's like learning to ride a bike. You can't just hop on and ride. You have to learn how to center yourself so you don't fall over.

The same is true with masturbation. Female orgasms are highly personal. They don't necessarily come naturally or easily. You have to be willing to explore how your own body works so that you can orgasm during masturbation and when you are with your partner.

(Side note: Just as some women still feel the need for feminine hygiene products, one of the major myths about sex is that women will orgasm from penile thrusting alone. It's just not true. No matter how hard or artfully your partner goes at it, at least half of women will never orgasm that way. That's because female orgasm has little to do with the vagina and everything to do with the clitoris, which usually needs direct, rhythmic stimulation...and which is not located inside the vagina.)

That said—and this is an extremely important point—I am not advocating that women masturbate all the time, either.

Here's a case in point: Vibrators are like magic buttons for clitoral stimulation, and that's why women love them for masturbation and as sex toys used with partners. A vibrator's strength isn't the issue; it'll either make you happy or it won't. Ideally, what you want the vibrator to do is keep you happy when you aren't able to have sex with your partner (for example, when one of you is traveling) or to help you learn more precisely what kinds of motions or stimulation turn you on the best.

But—and here's another one of those *big* buts—I am actually not a fan of vibrators or other sex toys for female masturbation because they do the same thing to women that chronic masturbation does to men. This is one of the big disagreements I have with sex therapists, who often tell women to use a vibrator if they don't have an orgasm easily.

That might be okay for women who aren't sexually active but still want the pleasures of masturbation. But I don't think that's good advice for those who *are* sexually active, because the ultimate goal is for them to have orgasms with their partners, not their sex toys. The vibrator is so good at stimulating the clitoris that if you use it regularly, you may soon become unable to orgasm without it. That means you may be left unsatisfied during sex with your partner, and who wants that?

The goal with any sexual relationship is to enjoy it together, not to enjoy *yourself* more than the relationship. If you are enjoying your hands-on experience too much, you have to figure out how to make a change-up or do it less frequently, just as men need to vary their masturbation techniques or use them less regularly to be less dependent on them.

For instance, if you take a long time to orgasm, you can start masturbating as part of your foreplay and then have your partner join in while he's getting ready to do his thing. This can give you both the satisfying experience you're hoping for. And when you know what stimulates you and gives you the greatest pleasure, have a hands-on experience with your partner, directing his fingers or his mouth. Show him how to move them the way you move your own fingers. Demonstrate what positions work best. Most of all have lots of fun and laughter doing so.

Trust me; the sex life you save will be your own!

The U.S. Food and Drug Administration has approved only two products for OTC treatment of premature ejaculation. One is a lidocaine spray that's available as a "male desensitizing" spray. The user has to spray it on his penis, rub it in, and then wait five to ten minutes for it to take effect. The other is benzocaine, an ingredient used in a liquid formulation for toothaches and also as a topical anesthetic. Again, it has to be rubbed on and then a man has to wait for five to ten minutes for it to work, but it's easier to use than the lidocaine spray. (These products have no adverse effects for women having sex with men using them—except, perhaps, in affecting your ready-for-it-now mood!)

To help men out, I've created the first benzocaine application in a wipe, called PreBoost (www.preboost.com). It can be applied easily and I consider it the most efficient way to not only treat premature ejaculation, but also to help these men enhance the sexual experience, at least long enough for their partners to be satisfied.

Dear Dr. Fisch: Can Kegel Exercises Help Me with My Premature Ejaculation?

Dear Dr. Fisch,

No matter what, I can't last more than a minute or so when I'm having sex. I read online that Kegel exercises can help. Is this true or just an Internet myth?

Signed, Frustrated

Dear Frustrated,

I don't blame you for feeling that way, as the average man has sex for five to ten minutes. But premature ejaculation is the number one cause of sexual dysfunction in men, and at one time or another, half of all men have to deal with it.

I wish I could say Kegel exercises could help you, but they can't. These exercises contract and relax the pelvic-floor muscles. They help women who have stress incontinence but don't do anything for a man's penis.

Juicy Fruit: Lubrication for Women

We've talked about men's ejaculation issues, so now it's time to turn to women. As you probably know, when a woman is sexually aroused, the walls of her vagina secrete a clear, slippery fluid that facilitates intercourse. As with everything else about humans, there is a fairly wide range of normal for vaginal lubrication. Some women produce lubrication easily and copiously, while others take longer and produce a lot less.

Staying "wet" is actually a big problem for many women. A study published in the February 2013 issue of the *Journal of Sexual Medicine* reported that 95 percent of women don't have enough lubrication to last during an entire lovemaking session, especially one that takes place over an extended time. (I was *shocked* when I saw that high number—and it takes a lot to shock me!) At some point, women may become dry. This can take sex from wonderful to "Whoa, stop." It can really hurt. Who wants to have sex when it's causing them pain?

Lack of lubrication also affects women in other ways. It is one of the most common causes of sexual dysfunction in women. If you're too dry, you'll never have an orgasm because your clitoris will not be able to get the stimulation it needs. It just gets dry, painful friction instead. In addition, dryness can lead to vaginal irritation, vaginal infections, and urinary tract infections, none of which are good for your health—or your sex life.

Vaginal dryness can be caused by genetic factors and by hormones, especially during pregnancy, childbirth, and nursing. During perimenopause (the time just before menopause starts) and menopause, natural lubrication decreases as well. Dryness can also be caused by emotional stress, unresolved issues between you and your partner, certain medications (such as some anti-histamines, antidepressants, and anti-anxiety drugs), and use of personal-care products such as bubble bath, scented soaps and lotions, and douching, all of which can disrupt the natural chemistry of the vagina.

Women think that they have to endure this extremely common situation, but there is no reason to suffer. If you're not getting wet enough, take action! Luckily, a woman's lubrication problem is almost always easy and inexpensive to remedy. Estrogen is one form, but it's not preferred. Although estrogen can help ease vaginal dryness, lots of women don't want to use hormone-based treatments because they are worried about the sometimes potent side effects of these treatments, especially after menopause. (The risk of these possible effects must, of course, be discussed with your gynecologist.)

The easiest solution to vaginal dryness is to use a high-quality lubricant, both for sex and to ease day-to-day dryness. Remember, though, that any type of personal lubricant can interfere with sperm and make it a lot harder to get pregnant. If you are trying to get pregnant, you may want to use natural lubricants such as canola oil or egg whites. Here are some tips for resolving dryness:

- Look for water-based lubricants, like the well-known K-Y Jelly (or other brands like Astroglide). If the brand you bought doesn't work well—some can dry out quickly or might not be slippery enough for you—try a different one.
- If your partner uses latex condoms, avoid all oil-based lubricants, as oil can wreak havoc on latex, weakening the condom and causing leaks or even breakage. Oil-based lubricants can also stain and be difficult to wash off. This means that petroleum jelly, mineral oil (such as baby oil), most hand lotions or body creams, and Marlon Brando's favorite (butter) in the infamous *Last Tango in Paris* are off the list.
- Speaking of condoms, look for lubricated brands. They can help a lot, too. Don't be shy about needing them. Incorporate their use into your sex play and foreplay with your partner. For example, you can sweetly tease your partner by opening the packet very slowly and continue with a teasing manner by even more slowly helping him to put it on properly.

Here are two other tips for communicating with your partner about this:

- Speak up if lubrication becomes an issue. It's totally normal.
- Know what's right for your needs. Keep a container of lube near the bed, and don't be shy about using it. Most women

say they want more lubrication rather than less. Needing this kind of product is completely normal and nothing to be ashamed about. After all, if more lubrication will help you orgasm, you'll enjoy sex more and probably want to have it more, too. Better sex leads to more sex!

Lubricating Warming Gel to Slow Down Men and Speed Up Women

So many men (and women) come to me frustrated about their or their partner's premature ejaculation problems that I decided to create an over-the-counter lubrication gel, called PreBoost Lubricating Warming Gel, to address both of their needs simultaneously (www.preboost.com). The goal is to help men who only last a short time to last longer and to help women who had trouble becoming stimulated to do so more quickly.

The gel's active ingredients are niacin, arginine (an amino acid), ginseng, and vitamin E. The gel absorbs extremely quickly, reducing the time needed to apply it and wait for it to start working. For men, the ingredients in the gel work by lessening friction during sex. For women, they work synergistically to warm the area, which keeps it moist and speeds up blood flow. Hopefully, products like this can help men and women achieve the satisfying sex they deserve.

Too Late: Inability to Orgasm

As you read earlier, premature ejaculation is often caused by chronic masturbation. In this section I'll discuss a related problem: a man's inability to ejaculate at all when he's having sex with his partner because of masturbation.

Susanna and her boyfriend, Brendan, have been in a relationship for nearly two years. In that time, he has been able to ejaculate only three times. He has been able to have an erection and get close to ejaculating, but then it won't happen unless he masturbates. Susanna is worried he may have a serious problem and has no idea what she can do to help.

"Susanna, I really hope you're not blaming yourself for this, because this is not your issue," I told her when she and Brendan showed up in my office. "Brendan is doing something that's unbelievably common."

I turned to Brendan. "I'll bet you have no trouble having an orgasm when you masturbate, right?"

"Right," he said.

"I'm glad," I said, "because it means there's no medical reason that might impede your ability to ejaculate, and you won't need any testing or have to worry about something being really wrong. What you have is called 'retarded ejaculation.' You've gotten so good at masturbating that your body has forgotten how to derive pleasure directly from you having sex with your partner. You can only achieve orgasm by using your own hand."

Brendan looked a little sheepish, so I quickly added, "I always say that masturbation isn't a problem unless it's hurting the relationship. In this case, though, that's what's going on. When men masturbate constantly, they develop what's called 'idiosyncratic masturbation,' where they're only able to achieve orgasm when they touch themselves in a very specific way. So you both can have some fun and start experimenting."

Susanna and Brendan looked at each other and smiled.

"First, Brendan needs to show you exactly how he masturbates to orgasm during foreplay," I said to Susanna. "That will give you an idea of the kind of stimulation he's used to. You may be able to mimic those rhythms or patterns during lovemaking, or by doing something similar with your hands to get him going.

"You can suggest that he tone down the masturbation and do it a lot less frequently. He can also change the way he masturbates and vary his technique. For example, if he always does it in the shower, stop using that location. If he only uses his right hand, try it with his left. If he doesn't ejaculate for a few days, he will become much more sensitive to stimulation. This should, by itself, raise the probability that he'll have an orgasm during lovemaking.

"Brendan, if you're comfortable with this approach, and you're both relaxed enough to try different things, I think you'll soon find that your sex life will improve tremendously."

Happily, Brendan called about a month later to tell me that he was having so much fun in bed with Susanna that he'd kicked his masturbation habit. I'd given them a lot of ideas about switching things up, and they tried all of them.

So if this is a problem for your partner, show him this section and use it to start a conversation. Or drop my suggestions into a conversation with your partner. You can say something like, "I'd love to have a 'naughty' weekend with you, so if you keep your hands off for a few days before then, I promise you the sexual experience of a lifetime." What man wouldn't want to go for that?

Performance Anxiety

Leonardo da Vinci was brilliant at a lot of things. He was certainly brilliant at understanding the male penis when he said: "Many times the man wishes it to practice and it does not wish it; many times it wishes it and the man forbids it."

Women can fake an orgasm with varying degrees of effectiveness (not that I'm advocating you *should* fake, of course!), but a penis is either visibly and physically hard and erect…or it isn't. At one time or another, all men will lose their erection just when they want it most. In this section, I'm not talking about premature ejaculation or lack of ejaculation due to chronic masturbation, but for other reasons: overuse of alcohol or drugs, too much stress, tension, exhaustion, distraction, depression, new partner worries (Will she like me?), an extended time since the last ejaculation, and even boredom. Many prescription medications can interfere with erections as well.

Physiologically, an erection arises (sorry, bad pun!) from a combination of male anatomy, hydraulics, chemistry, and nerve impulses. (Doesn't sound very sexy when you think about it that way, does it?) When it works, and works well, sex can be one of the best feelings in the world for him.

Unfortunately, what starts out as a purely physical phenomenon can do a real number on the male psyche when erections fail, setting up men for a vicious cycle of anxiety about getting erect and subsequent failure. And that cycle can do a real number on your ability to have a satisfying sex life. What began as a problem that can happen to any man at any time can quickly morph into a complicated psychological reaction called "performance anxiety."

Whenever a man has anxiety, his hormones send out signals to clamp down his blood vessels, including those feeding the penis. If he's afraid he won't be able to get it up and keep it up, he will create a self-fulfilling prophecy in which he physically can't, leaving him worried about sex (and having less sex), as well as feeling ashamed, angry, and abandoned.

Fortunately, many cases of performance anxiety can be alleviated by simply talking openly about the problem with your partner and helping him relax. Some men find that distraction or relaxation techniques can also help them keep their erection or delay ejaculation. Some men also need to abstain from smoking, recreational drugs, and drinking, as those can interfere with the ability to have and sustain an erection.

Make it clear to your partner that you know how normal it is to lose an erection once in a while, and that it's not about his masculinity or your attractiveness. It can happen to any man at any time, for all the reasons you just read about. Almost all of these men have *no idea* how common this problem is. If they did, I don't think it would upset them so much. The more you both can normalize it, and the less you both take it seriously, the quicker his erections—and sexual satisfaction for both of you—will come back.

Dear Dr. Fisch: Dating after Divorce Is Tough on Me and on My Erections

Dear Dr. Fisch,

I'm sixty-two, and after being married for eleven years, I got a divorce about a year ago. My ex-wife and I had a good sex life until our marriage fell apart, and I'm in good health, luckily, with no heart disease or high blood pressure or anything like that. I still get morning erections nearly every day. I'm now dating a woman who's fifty-seven, and we like each other a lot. I'm pretty sure she's going to want to have sex with me for the first time on our next date, and I'm worried that I might not perform well. What can I do to maintain a healthy erection?

Signed, Will I Get It Up?

Dear Will I Get It Up,

If you have an erection when you wake up in the morning, your plumbing is fine. Erectile dysfunction is different in people with health problems, just like it's different in younger versus older people. You would know if you couldn't get a healthy erection. So even though you're sixty-two, consider yourself lucky that you're like a twenty-six-year-old in bed!

In younger men, erectile dysfunction tends to be stress-related. You're worried about your new relationship the way a young man would be. Also, although wearing a condom decreases sensation, you must always use one until you know all of the health details about a new sexual partner. So performance anxiety and condoms are your issues.

If you know your partner's background or don't need to use a condom with her for some reason, or both, you may not have any problem. Since you have morning erections, try to have sex in the morning rather than at night if you use a condom. In the morning, your stress level will be lower, too.

If that doesn't work and you find yourself still anxious, you might want to take a break from sex for a while and deal with your anxieties, perhaps through short-term cognitive therapy. For serious anxiety-related sexual dysfunction, you should see a urologist to rule out any medical conditions and then discuss the option of taking medications like Viagra, Levitra, or Cialis, which tend to work well by helping to increase the blood flow to your penis.

Most of all relax and have fun!

You'd Be Amazed How Many Guys under Forty Can't Get It Up

Erectile dysfunction brings to mind the stereotype of an older man who's too pooped to pop, but many younger men (under forty) also have serious erection problems. Not all men are sexually confident studs who can go all night and then some. Lots of them worry about being in bed with a woman of short acquaintance, for example, or one they really like and want to impress. Erectile dysfunction not only can be a source of embarrassment for one or both partners, but also can lead to future anxiety that makes the problem worse.

Sometimes men feel emasculated or frustrated by their partners but don't know how to express this without hurting the woman they love. This was Connor's problem. He was thirty-two and engaged to a kindergarten teacher named Emily. They were happily planning the wedding and looking forward to their life together, but he confessed to me that Emily tended to treat him like one of her students in bed. She used babyish talk, bossed him around, and expected an immediate response to whatever she demanded. This led to a rather lackluster sexual response from him.

"It's nearly impossible to enjoy sex when you don't feel empowered during the experience," I told Connor. "Emily is treating you like a child in the bedroom, and most men wouldn't react to well to this."

I walked him through the need to communicate with his fiancée and how to do that. After our appointment, he was finally able to talk about what was going on in the bedroom, and Emily listened. Eventually sex became much more enjoyable and adult for him—and for Emily.

Connor's kind of performance anxiety was easily treatable without medication. The good news for young men with other kinds of performance anxiety is that Viagra and other similar drugs work phenomenally well in short stints. And younger men don't have to worry about becoming dependent on these drugs because once they get going and realize they *can* get going and keep going, they don't need meds anymore. Their performance anxiety is gone.

For much more information about erection meds, turn to page 109 in Lesson 3.

Dear Dr. Fisch: As Soon as I Lost My Job, I Lost My Erection

Dear Dr. Fisch,
I lost my job a couple of months ago, and I've lost my mojo. My wife works long hours to keep us afloat. I

can stay hard when I'm masturbating, but not when I'm having sex with my wife. How can I feel confident again?
  Signed, Lost My Mojo

Dear Lost My Mojo,
  I'm sure you're going through a very stressful period in your life, especially when your wife has become the primary breadwinner in your household. This can be a blow to a man's ego. Having performance anxiety is a very common problem for men, especially when they are going through rough times.
  You may be masturbating, in part, as a release or escape from the stresses and feelings surrounding your job loss and subsequent role-reversal. That's fairly normal—and a whole lot better than using drugs or alcohol to blunt the worries—but you're not dealing with these issues directly. While self-stimulation releases endorphins that temporarily ease pain and elevate mood, it can also act as a drug of sorts, distracting you from focusing on what you need to be doing right now to improve your situation. So I'm advising you to stop masturbating because I know you'd rather have a relationship with your wife than with your hand!
  While you're working on getting another job, focus on the woman who loves you. All these issues should be discussed openly so that you two can share the worries honestly. That alone may reduce your anxiety so your sexual performance with your wife improves.

If that doesn't help, you might want to consider short-term use of a medication to treat erectile dysfunction while you're living with so much stress. For most of my patients, when the anxiety and stressful situations leading to performance anxiety are lessened or gone, sexual problems also decrease or disappear.

It's Not Surprising How Many Men over Forty Can't Keep It Up

Being able to quickly respond to and no longer need drugs like Viagra is the difference between the performance anxiety of a younger man and an older one. As testosterone levels drop, so does the penis. I call it "the angle of the dangle." This refers to the fact that how high a man's erection juts out from his body indicates his age. Hold your hand perpendicular to your chest with the inside of your wrist facing your chest. Your thumb will be like a man in his twenties. The pinkie is a man in his sixties. It's the same thing for an erection. You get the picture!

But there is no reason for any man to suffer (often in silence) and worry about his ability to have a satisfying sex life. Having aging male patients ask for Viagra allows me to candidly discuss their other health issues and refer them to other specialists if they need them. In a way, it's as if Viagra has brought people out of the closet for treatment of other medical conditions that affect their sex lives, such as weight issues, diabetes, high blood pressure, and heart disease. (For more information about treating sexual dysfunction, see page 87 in Lesson 3.)

Sometimes, performance anxiety has nothing to do with the ability to have and maintain erections, as Wayne found out. He's fifty-five and has been married to Christine for thirty years. Their kids are grown and out of the house.

"I thought we were happy together. We had a normal sex life, I guess," Wayne said to me, his brow furrowed as he toyed nervously with a pen. "But lately, she's been acting all different in the bedroom and she's starting to scare me. I think she's cheating on me and trying to get out of our marriage."

"What does she say when you ask her about this?" I said.

"She says she's just trying to make me happy 'cause the kids are gone. She wants to have more fun and go out more, like when we were first dating. And she wants to play around a lot more in bed. I don't know what to do!"

Ah. Wayne's performance anxiety had nothing to do with his physical ability to have sex. Instead, he was riddled with insecurities about his relationship with his wife.

"What I'm hearing is that the sex life you've had for years is suddenly not good enough for your wife anymore. You don't understand where this could be coming from, so you're taking it personally.

"But if you listen to your wife, you'll understand that this isn't what she's telling you," I went on. "You're very fortunate that your wife wants to connect with you again physically. It's not unreasonable to try and spice up a sex life. This is completely normal and happens a lot in women, especially as they get older and their hormone levels change. She doesn't have to worry about getting pregnant or the kids barging into the room in the middle of the night. She just wants to be with *you*!"

I told Wayne to ask Christine to explain exactly what she wants in the bedroom. She might be worried that he didn't find her attractive or desirable anymore. If she wanted to try out different positions in the bedroom, they should talk about it beforehand and figure out a sexual style that they're both comfortable with.

"And most of all don't be scared of trying new things that keep you two having fun in bed."

Wayne looked a lot less worried when he left.

LESSON 2

WHAT TURNS YOU OFF TO SEX?

I s it easier to get turned on or turned off?

Or, said another way, what turns you off to sex?

I deal with this topic every day in my office and with callers to my radio show who are looking for sex and relationship answers. We all know that sex is more than just hormonal urges or a perpetuate-the-species biological drive to go forth and make lots of babies. Sex is an integral part of life and especially of healthy relationships. Our sexual drive, or libido, is as hardwired into our systems as breathing, sleeping when we're tired, stopping to eat when we're hungry, seeking a purpose in life (in other words, a satisfying career), and experiencing the joys of love from friends and family.

Our libido is also in constant flux due to the stresses of daily life, the demands of pregnancy and child rearing, our health, our feelings of trust and intimacy with our partners, and even our sense of familiarity or boredom, or both, with these same partners.

But no matter what's going on in your life, the number one reason people get turned off to sex is that it's just not fun for them. The number two reason is because our partner has pissed us off, and we just don't want to get close at the moment (or potentially for a while afterward).

Let's be realistic: expecting two people to have the same libido at the same moment of every day might be ideal but often isn't feasible, as much as you might wish it were. At some point or another, everyone is going to have one of those days, weeks, or maybe even longer, when they're just not in the mood.

There could be any number of valid reasons: a newborn baby leaving you so tired you want to glue your legs shut for the next decade; too much work leaving you utterly drained at the end of the day; monthly cramps that make you wish you could inject chocolate directly into your abdomen to make the annoying pains go away; or your partner in a bad mood, which pisses you off and makes you want to throttle, not embrace, him or her. That, in turn, can escalate into devastating fights. Fighting can also be triggered when your partner doesn't listen, when you're chronically ignored, or when you feel like you're being patronized or dismissed.

You know, *life* gets in the way. But so does ignorance.

Remember, it's not what happens in the bedroom that affects your sex life; it's everything that happens *before* you get into the bedroom. And this can cause a lot of tension between partners.

If sex is fabulous fun and makes you feel good, especially with a partner you love, then you're going to have a lot of regular sex. It's like exercise. You know you need it, and you know it'll make you feel good because your body needs it. The more you have, the better you feel. Having regular, satisfying sex is an integral component of any strong relationship. So whatever the reason, when the sex slows to a crawl, it's time to take action.

What If He Won't Have Sex with Me?

If your sex life is going through a bad patch, don't jump to the conclusion that something dire is happening, and don't take it as a personal affront or rejection. Yes, your partner could be having an affair, but more likely he's having a bad time at work and doesn't want to share all the horrible details with you. (And no, he's not sharing the details or a bed with anyone else.)

Yes, it's possible he could be going to prostitutes because he doesn't know anything about the physical causes of sexual dysfunction, but more likely his testosterone levels are so low they've squashed his libido flatter than his hair on a rainy day. Sure, there is a remote chance he might be clinically depressed, but more likely he's just going through a phase where he's worried about aging or feeling insecure for some reason.

Let's take a look at some of the primary reasons why sex has slowed, and then you can take a quiz for each category to determine what the issue might be.

- He's cheating. (For the quiz and more information, go to Lesson 4, starting on page 129.)
- He's unusually stressed.
- He's depressed.
- He's got low testosterone.
- He's gay and in the closet.
- He's addicted to porn. (For the quiz and more information, go to Lesson 4, starting on page 129.)

QUIZ

IS HE UNUSUALLY STRESSED?

- ☐ Have his sleep patterns changed?
- ☐ Has he had drastic changes in his weight?
- ☐ Is he exhausted all the time?
- ☐ Does he have trouble concentrating?
- ☐ Does his skin tone seem ashy or different?
- ☐ Does he seem unusually nervous or anxious?
- ☐ Is he moody, or moodier than usual?
- ☐ Does he frequently seem unhappy or sad, or both?
- ☐ Does he get a lot of phone calls from work or from family members, and do these phone calls seem to stress, aggravate, or worry him?
- ☐ Does he talk about getting away from it all?
- ☐ Does he snap at you when you want to talk?
- ☐ Or does he tell you everything's fine when you know it's not?
- ☐ Is he drinking more than usual?

How Can You Tell If He's Unusually Stressed?

Stress can take its toll in all sorts of ways. If they have the energy, some men want to have lots of sex as a release for all the tension they're dealing with. Other men are the complete opposite. They withdraw and withhold.

If your partner is going through tough times due to problems at work, with family (your immediate family or other relatives), with friends, or with himself, you've got to communicate. Getting a man to open up can be really hard when he's used to being stoic or tight-lipped. But if he holds it all in, the stress might get worse, leading to depression, substance abuse (to help deal with the feelings of failure or being out of control of managing the situation), or further withdrawal. For more on depression, see the next section—and remember that stress is not the same as depression but can be a contributing factor. For specific tips on how to communicate effectively with a stressed-out partner and how to support him, read on to Part II.

Remember: a burden shared is a burden lessened. Get him to talk, however you can!

Dear Dr. Fisch: My Wife and I Are Working Too Much and It's Taking Its Toll

Dear Dr. Fisch,

My wife and I are both thirty, and we've been married for two years. We're both under a lot of strain at work, with long hours and a lot of stress. Things just aren't the way they used to be. We hardly have sex any more, and when we do, there's no more spark and fun like we used to have. And when I told my wife that I was going to either call your radio show or make an appointment to see you, she got so mad she stormed out of the house. I don't know what to do.

Signed, Work Sucks

Dear Work Sucks,

I'm sorry to hear this. The fact that your wife stormed out isn't a great sign, but she may have just lost it because she's as stressed out or exhausted as you are. You know how easy that reaction is, especially when you're feeling overwhelmed by your current predicament. Problems at work leading to stress and exhaustion can certainly send sex flying out the window. But that should only be temporary.

It seems like you two could communicate better. From your wife's reaction to your attempted solution, it's fairly clear that you're not communicating effectively about how your stress at work and your job schedules are making you both miserable—and you're definitely not communicating about sex. I'll bet your exhaustion keeps you from being able to talk candidly.

The fact that you're reaching out to me signals that you already recognize how unhealthy it is to let your sexual relationship dwindle. Having a good sex life is one of the most important things in a quality relationship, especially for young couples who haven't been married long. Sex can actually alleviate a lot of the stress you're dealing with, because it's physically relaxing and will bring you together on a deeper, more intimate level.

You need to ask yourself if there's something more than just exhaustion going on here. At this point, sex should not be the first thing on your mind. Obviously, she stormed out because she's very angry about something, and you'll need to find out what that is. When you know she's not so tired or frustrated, say to her gently, "I really love you, and I really miss how good our sex life was. What can we start doing as a team to get things working again? What can I do to make you enjoy having sex more?"

See what she says and take it from there. Do not keep things bottled up, because it's crucial to get to the root of her anger right now. I guarantee that if you give her the space and listen so that she can tell you exactly what she wants from you—and you do it!—then you two will end up having better sex *and* a much better relationship.

I've said this many times but it's worth repeating: It's not just what happens in the bedroom that affects your sex life, it's everything that happens outside the bedroom, too.

IS HE DEPRESSED?

☐ Has he shown a loss of interest in usual activities that engage him?

☐ Is his libido nonexistent?

☐ Has his depressed mood lasted longer than two weeks?

☐ Are you having frequent fights without any resolution?

☐ Is he unusually anxious?

☐ Is he unable to do the simple tasks he usually did without any problems?

☐ Is he having trouble concentrating?

☐ Have his sleep patterns changed (such as difficulty falling asleep or staying asleep, early-morning awakening, sleeping more than usual)?

☐ Has his appetite changed?

☐ Has he gained or lost a lot of weight suddenly?

☐ Is he drinking more or taking drugs?

☐ Is he avoiding friends?

☐ Is he unwilling to talk?

☐ Does he shut himself away in his room or another part of the house?

☐ Does he blow off things that used to make him happy?

☐ Is he feeling more pessimistic?

☐ Does he admit he feels worthless?

☐ Is he unusually bitter or angry?

☐ Has he mentioned wanting to die or suicide?

How Can You Tell If He's Depressed?

It is incredibly frustrating to me that mental illnesses are still such a source of shame and mistreatment in this country. If you get cancer, you wouldn't hesitate to get it treated, right? But if you—and especially if men—get a brain-based illness such as anxiety or depression, drumming up the courage to seek help, let alone *good* help, can be a lot harder. Finding a therapist isn't always easy or covered by insurance.

Admitting that you're feeling bad isn't easy for either men or women. But since women tend to be more in touch with emotional realities—and men more prone to bottling them up, women are more likely to seek out a medical professional, such as a psychologist or psychiatrist, for counseling.

A man who's depressed needs help. As long as his depression goes untreated, his libido is shot (unless he is diagnosed as bipolar, in which case he might want a tremendous amount of sex in a manic phase, and none at all when he's crashing into sadness). The quiz lists many of the markers for depression, and if you want more advice, speak to your physician or your own therapist about your worries and see if he or she can provide referrals or ideas for further treatment. You can also research different options at a trusted web source such as WebMD (www.webmd.com/depression/guide/depression-resources).

It's not easy to broach the subject—which is why "How to Bring Up a Delicate Topic" (on page 195 in Lesson 5) can help—but a man who is depressed has an illness that needs immediate medical care from a competent therapist. Low-level depression can respond to exercise, meditation, dietary changes, and short-term therapy, without any medication needed. Chronic depression, on the other hand, is an extremely serious illness that is nearly impossible to lift without professional support. Help your man seek help. When appropriate, prescribed medication treatments, such as antidepressants, can be lifesavers for both your man's mood and your relationship.

IS HE SUFFERING FROM LOW TESTOSTERONE?

☐ Is he tired all the time?
☐ Is he having erection problems?
☐ Is his sleep constantly disrupted or not deep enough to make him feel rested?
☐ Has he lost his sexual spark?
☐ Does he just not want to have sex anymore?
☐ Does he have low muscle tone?
☐ Are his testicles small or soft?
☐ Has he gained weight, particularly around his waist?
☐ Has he been diagnosed with osteoporosis?
☐ Has he been diagnosed with anemia?
☐ Is he depressed?
☐ Does he tell you he just feels blah without knowing why?

How Can You Tell If He Has Low Testosterone?

Low testosterone equals a low libido. In this case, he needs to see a doctor and have a complete blood workup. There's no reason to suffer from this when it is so easy to treat!

For lots more information about low testosterone levels and what to do about them, see page 87 in Lesson 3.

IS HE GAY AND STILL IN THE CLOSET?

- ☐ Are you having significantly less sex over a long period of time?
- ☐ Does he get defensive when you bring up your sex life?
- ☐ Is he blaming you for any sexual problems?
- ☐ Does he suddenly want you to use sex toys to stimulate him, particularly sex toys than involve anal penetration, such as a strap-on dildo or vibrators?
- ☐ Is he unusually secretive about phone calls or email or his social life?
- ☐ Does he hide his computer history from you?
- ☐ Have you found him looking at gay porn?
- ☐ Has he replied to any gay online dating sites?
- ☐ Does he look at men (instead of women) a little bit too long, as if he's checking them out?
- ☐ Does he tell you he's going to gay bars with his friends who are gay, but he's "not"?
- ☐ Is he moody or angry at you for no reason?
- ☐ Is he more interested than usual in his appearance?
- ☐ Is he spending an inordinate amount of time at the gym or working out?
- ☐ Does he go on trips "with the guys" and not allow you to meet them?

How Can You Tell If He's Gay and Still in the Closet?

A man who is gay is naturally programmed to be with other men sexually, not with women. If he is living a lie for whatever reason, at some point he probably will not want to have sex with you.

Gay men get married to straight women for reasons such as a need for security and a fear of being alone; genuine affection; or an inability to come to grips with their true sexual orientation, often coupled with deep denial and even deeper fear of being "exposed," often as a result of being reared in a home where homosexuality was thought of as evil, sinful, unnatural, or degrading.

Most women who marry gay men do so when they want to be in a relationship so badly that they're willing to overlook a lot of signs that point to the man's sexual orientation. It's often easy for women to become close to and develop a passionate love for gay men who can give them the emotional connection they seek and haven't always gotten from heterosexual partners.

Believe me, I am not being judgmental when I say I think that most women I've seen whose partners are gay know deep down that they are. In retrospect, some of the signs were there. If you know this and the relationship works for you, and you're both happy, I say more power to you. However, I don't think that most couples who are living in such denial can sustain that happiness over a lifetime.

Here's one rather extreme example I witnessed in my office. The reasons why Brendan and Lucinda came to see me spilled out quickly. Brendan was suffering from premature ejaculation, and Lucinda admitted that she was toying with the idea of bringing another woman into their relationship to spice up their sex life. (Not exactly what I'd call a realistic plan.) I immediately had a feeling there was a lot more to this story than what they had told me.

"Well, Lucinda, since Brendan isn't satisfying you, you think bringing in another woman could liven up your relationship. You need to tell Brendan what you want in the bedroom that would satisfy your desires, while still communicating your love for him in that fantasy. So what do you need Brendan to do to make sex more satisfying for you?"

Brendan interrupts. "Do I need to bring another man in?"

There it was. I knew exactly how this conversation was going to end.

"No! Of course not!" Lucinda said, looking shocked. "I don't want another man in the bedroom with us. Having a threesome with another woman is my fantasy. And if you're interested in other women, this way we can both have fun."

Brendan frowned. "I don't want to do that. I might be interested in dating another man… I've been having these feelings for men lately."

Lucinda looked even more shocked.

"Lucinda," I said gently, "think about how you just reacted when Brendan said he wanted to be with another man. I think you now understand how he felt when you said you wanted to be with another woman. Do you really want to do that, or are you looking for ways to get Brendan more interested in sex again?"

"But this is the first time Brendan has said anything like that. I can't believe it," she added, on the verge of tears. "At least he already knew about my fantasies. I haven't acted on them or anything like that. I honestly don't know if I could, anyway. And now he's telling me he wants to have sex with a man."

"Brendan, do you really want to have sex with another man?" I asked him. "Have you had sex with another man?"

Brendan looked only a little sheepish—not because having sex with men is wrong, but because he was about to not only admit to cheating but to being gay.

"Yes, I have. Lucinda, honestly, I'm really sorry. I am. I've been having oral sex with another man."

Lucinda burst into tears. "For how long?"

"For about two months," Brendan confessed. "For as long as I haven't been able to ejaculate with you. I'm sorry."

"Go on," I prompted.

"Lucinda, I'm gay," he said. "I've been wanting to tell you for a long time, but I didn't want to hurt your feelings. I love men. It's over. I want to move on, and I need to move out. I'm sorry, but I have to."

This wasn't the most tactful way to drop such a bombshell on a loving wife, was it? Lucinda became distraught, and their marriage was irrevocably shattered.

Not every couple dealing with a similar, albeit less extreme situation will see the relationship end, of course. As I said already, some couples work it out and are content with their sexual and emotional lives. What makes these relationships work is loving honesty about each other's needs and desires.

If you're wondering how to broach the topic, it might be helpful to use a neutral third party, such as a marital counselor or trusted advisor. There is no easy way to deal with this. You have to ask the question and jump in the pool, even though you know the water is cold. A supportive therapist or counselor will help ask the delicate questions and give you strategies for moving forward.

Dear Dr. Fisch: Is My Husband Gay?

Dear Dr. Fisch,

I'm really worried about my marriage. My husband and I have been married for ten years and we have two small children, but we haven't had sex in over six months. He used to steal my razors and shave off a lot of his leg hair, but one day he came home with nearly all his body hair—his chest hair and his pubic hair and even his facial hair—lasered off, and it's a huge turnoff for me. He looks like a baby, all smooth and pink. I can't believe he did this without discussing it with me first. I'm wondering, could he be gay? The last time I asked him, he left and didn't come back for three days.

Signed, Hiding the Razors

Dear Hiding the Razors,

I can't believe your husband got all his body hair removed, just like that! Talk about extreme. It's almost as extreme as women who get Brazilians because their partners tell them to. (And yes, I think women doing something they may not want to solely for a partner's pleasure can be extreme.)

I understand why this makes him less attractive and manly to you. Women are used to men having body hair. And you know what? Oils stick to body hair and give off a musky scent that a lot of women find sub-liminally alluring. The theory is that your body gives off pheromones, a scent that attracts the opposite sex.

That's one of the reasons why women wear perfume. They don't just want to smell good for themselves; they want to smell more attractive to men, too.

Anyway, it's clear that something else is going on. This is about more than just his hair, or lack thereof. I hate to tell you this, but your husband is being very narcissistic and treating you badly. It's likely he's either getting sex from someone else or having so much sex with himself that he's lost interest in you. But my inclination is that your husband could be having sex with other men, especially given his (for lack of a better word) extreme reaction, storming out the last time you asked him. A man who can answer "No" to that question doesn't leave.

At some point, you two need to have a very frank conversation, as hard as that might be. If you find the thought of that conversation untenable, you may want to find a good therapist so a neutral party can help frame the questions and help you both deal with the answers calmly. You and your relationship deserve it.

Dealing with the Consequences

So what do you do if you answered yes to some or many of the questions in a particular quiz? If you answered a strong yes to at least a few questions on any of them, you probably realize that you or your partner is likely in denial about one of these issues. You may even be feeling relieved because at least you know the truth or can take steps to get to the bottom of it.

Only you can decide whether you want to stay in your

relationship and see if you both can work things out. The goal of this book is to help you deal with the sexual issues and get to the truth of what's going on, good and bad, easy or tough. My advice in these situations is to find someone with compassion and understanding, whether a professional therapist or a trusted friend, to help guide and support you so you can make the best decisions for you and your relationship.

What If You Don't Want to Have Sex with Him?

Just as there are reasons why a man doesn't want to have sex with you, there are plenty of reasons why he might be turning you off. If any of the following hits close to home, it's time to start talking!

If He's Size XL But Not Where You Want Him to Be, It's Time to Lose the Weight

Obesity is at epidemic levels in this country, and men need to deal with the overeating and under-exercising that cause it if they want to live as long as possible and be healthy and thriving instead of fat and miserable.

I tell my patients that the goal isn't just to lose weight; it's to lose the waist. Because a man with a big, fat gut is pretty much guaranteed *not* to have big, fat testosterone levels and big, fat erections. (You'll read about this in more detail on page 93 of Lesson 3.)

Big, fat guts aren't just physical turnoffs for you; they're dangerous for a man's health. They'll reduce testosterone, which will make a man feel like crap, be tired all the time, and have a low libido. And a big, fat gut and excess weight elsewhere can cause too many diseases to name, all of which can have a terrible effect on his ability to have sex, as well as being off-putting for both of you.

A man who is obese can also develop "man boobs." For most women, it's a total turnoff if their male partners have a bigger breast size than they do. Of course, any man who isn't overweight but still has man boobs should see a doctor to rule out hormonal problems or other possible causes. If the cause is a medical condition, he can take meds to help reduce breast swelling or have liposuction or breast-reduction surgery if all else fails.

For more information about weight, see page 93 in Lesson 3. But in the meantime, tell him to lose the weight so your sex life will be great.

Dear Dr. Fisch: I Know I'm a Turnoff to Women. Help Me!

Dear Dr. Fisch,

I'm 32, 5'10", and weigh about 400 pounds. I'm single and I don't want to be, but I'm repulsed by my own body and I know that women are, too. But I can't stop eating and I'm too embarrassed and ashamed to get any exercise. How can I get over my addiction to food and find someone to love and who'll love me?

Signed, Too Tubby to Tango

Dear Too Tubby to Tango,

Food is delicious and makes you happy. I understand that. I love food, too, and I eat a lot, but I exercise more than anybody I know. You need to change your relationship with food drastically. I'm worried about your health, because you are at grave risk for serious diseases like diabetes, heart disease, strokes, or hypertension, which is high blood pressure.

Unless you are able to lose about 160 to 200 pounds, your risk will stay high and you will actually lower your life span. I do not want that to happen to you—and I'm sure you don't, either! You also may be having sexual difficulties because excess weight wreaks havoc on all parts of your body, no matter how much you want to have sex.

I understand that eating is your favorite habit and hobby, but in order to find and have a successful relationship, you first must find other activities besides food that make you happy. Relationships with other people could help—girl friends and guy friends both. Take up different hobbies and hang out with friends. (Hiding at home and playing games on the computer doesn't count.) Both will get you out of the house, distract you from wanting to eat all the time, and help you lose weight and meet women.

The more active you are, the more easily the weight will come off. To exercise, start by buying a pedometer at a local health store. Walk 10,000 steps a day, or the equivalent of about five miles, and the pounds will melt off. Try to get a workout buddy who'll keep you motivated. If you can afford it, hire a personal trainer to show you a routine that is safe and is something you like to do, which will help you stick with it. Of course, you need to speak to your doctor first to be sure you don't do anything too strenuous at first. Start slowly and when the pounds come off, it'll be easier to stay motivated.

As for diet: no breads, pizza, pasta, cookies, or cake. No added salt or sugar. Right now, these foods are not your friends. Find a good nutritionist or join a reputable group like Weight Watchers. You will not be judged; you will get out of the house to go to meetings; and you'll meet lots of women and make new friends.

One more tip: to decrease your appetite, drink water with lemon. Not lemonade. Just plain water with real lemon. Good luck! You can do it.

If His Grooming Is for the Dogs, Time for Him to Get His Shave On

A lot of men don't realize how important grooming and personal hygiene are to their partners, even though some women get turned on by guys who are, well, a little (okay, a *lot*!) on the ripe side. Unfortunately, women usually need to take the initiative to get guys to clean up their acts—and their bodies—and spruce up their sex lives in the process. Here are the top items to address on his grooming must-do list:

Shave

Stubble might look sexy, but his five o'clock shadow can leave your face looking and feeling like a Brillo pad after a lovemaking session. Not exactly the biggest turn-on.

There are two methods that usually work when you're trying to keep your skin intact. The first is to incorporate shaving into your foreplay. Don't make any moves that can end up with him getting nicked, but a little bit of pillow talk and perhaps some tender touching while a man is foaming up and then shaving can really get him in the mood.

If that doesn't work, or you telling him that shaving will lead to more romps in the bedroom, appeal to his vanity. Tell him that while shaving can be a chore, there's a hidden benefit to it for him (besides keeping your skin from shredding). Exfoliation. I don't expect this to be something men know much about, but they (and you) should.

As a natural part of the aging process, skin cells are born, come to the surface of your skin, and then die. This process slows down as you age, which is why your skin can look dull and blah. The shaving process, however, sloughs off those dead cells. This is one of the reasons why men's skin shows fewer signs of aging than women's. Hopefully this two-for-one deal will help him get his shave on.

Lather Up

Not just any soap. Deodorant soap. Every day. In the bath or shower. Lots of lather in the pubic area. Followed by deodorant.

Bear in mind that deodorants mask odor only, and antiperspirants help reduce sweat. If a man sweats excessively, so that even clinical antiperspirants don't do the job, he might be a good candidate for prescription deodorants or underarm Botox injections, which are amazingly efficient.

He also needs to clean his skin at night, just like you do. Who wants to go to bed with a face full of the day's grime? Of course you know that, but getting him to act on it can be as difficult as getting a toddler to sit still for an ear cleaning! So, as with shaving, try incorporating a nighttime de-griming ritual into your foreplay. Offer to wash his face if he'll wash yours. Give his face and his head a brief massage while you're at it. He'll have super-clean skin, and you'll both be laughing and relaxed. The rest is up to you!

Rinse and Repeat

Just as he needs to clean his skin, he needs to wash and condition his hair. Oily hair looks and smells gross. Dandruff is about as sexy as dust. Get into the shower with him and pour on some of your coconut-scented shampoo and pretend you're at the beach. If that doesn't get him in the mood, try a different scent!

Hydrate

A man's skin may seem to age less rapidly than yours, but that doesn't mean it's immune to the drying effects of getting older. He still needs to moisturize. Instead of letting him poach your products, show him the wide range of effective male skin-care lines. There are shelves of them at Sephora or at department stores, and he should experiment until he finds one with a scent, texture, and effectiveness he likes.

Protect

Skin cancers are on the rise, so sun protection is a must. An easy way to get a man to moisturize is to insist that he puts on sunscreen in the morning when you put yours on. Aim for an SPF of at least 25 to 30. Do not let him stash the bottle in the car, because sunscreen degrades in heat. (That's one of the reasons you need to keep reapplying it when you're out in the sun, especially at the beach!)

Conceal

Dark under-eye circles are, unfortunately, genetic, so as embarrassing as this might be for him (because most men would never dream of using this kind of product), show him how to use your own concealer. Convince him to try it by telling him that, as he likely knows already, men who *look* tired when they're not due to eye bags are unfairly judged as *being* tired. No one need ever know that he's using concealer, once you show him how to blend it in well. If that doesn't work well, he might want to consult a plastic surgeon to see if the dark circles can be removed. (Ditto with droopy eyelids.)

Many men also suffer from rosacea, an incurable and progressive skin condition leading to uncontrollable flushing. (Take a look at the comic movie star of the 1930s, W. C. Fields, for an example of extreme rosacea that also affected his nose.) This warrants a trip to the dermatologist. In the meantime, your man can try using a green-based foundation or primer that will help camouflage some of the redness.

Speaking of which, adult acne is a deeply embarrassing problem for a lot of men. While there are effective drugstore products for acne treatment, most are for teenagers, who tend to have much oilier skin. He should see a dermatologist first and discuss treatment options.

If His Closet Hasn't Had an Overhaul Since High School, He Needs a Makeover

When I was a resident in medical school, one of my fellow colleagues was a complete slob. He was such a mess that I had no confidence in his ability to make life-and-death decisions. He was working in a hospital, where cleanliness is of real concern and filth can be lethal. Patients never wanted to talk to him. So *we* all had a talk with him and directed him to the local Laundromat.

I'm not saying that a man needs a closet full of designer clothes. He doesn't. I've seen men look incredibly put together wearing nothing more than a crisply pressed white button-down shirt, a sleek leather belt, and a good-fitting pair of jeans. But he needs to look presentable. When I see my patients, I always wear a suit, a nice shirt, and a tie. My shoes are shined. I want them to see that I respect who *they* are by presenting myself in the best possible way. Other men should do the same.

I tell my patients to think of how they dress as part of foreplay. When you get a present all wrapped up in a gorgeous box with a bow, you get excited. It shows that someone cared enough to make that gift extra-special. If you get something covered in crumpled newspaper, or worse, just shoved at you with no ceremony at all, you're not nearly as likely to be enthusiastic and receptive.

Believe me: If a man doesn't look like he can take care of himself, you aren't going to think that he can take care of *you*.

If His Manners Are Lacking, So Probably Is Your Desire

Manners are one of those things where a tiny amount of effort can reap huge rewards. I always say that it's easy to be respectful and polite to the president of the United States, but how about the guy who cleans your office or parks your car? If I eat a meal I love at a restaurant, I want to meet the chef and the owner to say thank you. My wife and I always told our children that they don't have to like everybody they meet, but they have to be nice. Or try their best to be. It's not hard to be nice to somebody who doesn't expect it. What makes someone feel more desirable than a compliment?

Honestly, you can tell an awful lot about people by how they treat the help. When you're with a man with impeccable manners who is courteous and considerate to strangers, chances are good he's going to be that way in bed with you. Especially when he turns off the cell phone so he can concentrate on what's really important—namely you! (See the section on digital devices for more about that.)

If, on the other hand, he's rude or thoughtless or narcissistic, how is he going to treat you in the bedroom (let alone in a relationship), and why would you want to have sex with him? What a turnoff if he's in a bad mood and taking it out on you…or he dissed you in the morning, and you never got resolution…or he ignores you all evening until it's time for sex.

Even after you've been with your partner for years, there's no excuse for his lack of manners, or his making you feel that you're being taken for granted. You need to speak up. If he's been acting this way for a long time, he might not even be aware of what a problem it is, although of course that is no excuse. If you don't feel comfortable speaking up, this is an issue I suggest you bring up with a therapist, because allowing your partner to treat other people (and you) badly is indicative of deep-seated self-esteem issues that must be confronted in a safe and therapeutic setting.

If the Snoring Keeps You Awake, You'll Be Looking for the Checkout Hotel

Being unable to sleep because your partner's snores are louder than the disco drums in your favorite club is unlikely to put you in the mood for sex or cuddling or the wonderful intimacy that comes from sharing the same bed.

But snoring isn't just a case of buzz saws going off on the next pillow. Something has to be causing it. The reason could be relatively benign, like allergies, acid reflux, or large tonsils, or something more worrisome, like sleep apnea. Why should you or, more importantly, your partner worry about something like sleep apnea? Here's the catch: Sleep apnea is directly related to low testosterone (and a low libido). These two conditions are related to a man being overweight or not taking care of himself—and who wants to be with a man who cares so little about his health (and *your* ability to get to sleep)?

For more about snoring and sleep disorders, go to page 122 in Lesson 3. These problems need to be dealt with—not just so you can get your beauty rest, but because they can be signs of physical problems that can't self-heal and must be addressed. Sleep apnea is a dangerous condition and can, in fact, be lethal. And that would definitely mean no sex for you—or for him.

If He's Addicted to His Digital Devices, He Should Turn Them Off and Turn You On Instead

Have you watched people walk down the street in a big city lately? Are they striding confidently, heads held high, eyes on the horizon? Nope. Their heads are all bent down as they check their email and surf the Internet. Do they look strong, confident, sexy, and attractive? Nope. They look miserable, squinting with concentration as they peer at that all-too-important tiny, glowing screen for the latest text or email that, let's face it, can wait 99.9 percent of the time. I think the only people truly ecstatic about this terrible posture are the chiropractors and massage therapists hired to treat it.

In a few short years, our lives have become dominated by digital technology. As soon as the phone or computer or tablet chirps or beeps or otherwise lets us know that someone or something has communicated, we jump. I've had patients in my office who can't tear their eyes off their smartphones. At the risk of sounding old school, I've been at intimate dinner parties where people are so astonishingly rude that they answer a call in the middle of the salad course.

I've been disturbed in the theater and at the movies by people turning on their phones in the dark. I've had phone conversations where I can hear the surreptitious tap-tap-tap of a keyboard when I'm trying to make an important point. It's maddening, and it's not helping us have better lives, especially not better sex lives. In fact, a June 2013 survey by Harris Interactive found that nearly 20 percent of Americans age eighteen to thirty-four use their smartphones during sex, and nearly one in ten American adults overall uses them during sex. The survey didn't ask what the phones were used for. Porn viewing, maybe? Email checking, just as likely.

I find that absolutely astonishing—and terrifying. Who wants to make love to a phone? What kind of foreplay are you having if your partner is constantly on the phone or glued to a computer? How can he be "there" with you if his mind is elsewhere? It's impossible to be in the moment, right there with a real person, when you're tethered to virtual reality.

My advice is to set up bedroom rules for all digital devices. Whatever you do, keep them out of the bedroom when you're having sex. If you must use them during the rest of your quality time together, use them to engage the other person, such as sending a sexy text or showing a cute picture that will make him or her smile or laugh. Ultimately, turning your devices off will help turn you on.

LESSON 3

ERECTION, INTERRUPTED
THE ANATOMY OF SEXUAL DYSFUNCTION

In Lesson 1, I talked about how masturbation can wreak havoc on a man's ability to have a great sexual relationship with his partner, as well as the emotional issues behind performance anxiety. In this lesson, I'm going to tell you more about the physiological reasons for bad sex. I know how much misinformation is out there and believed even by educated and savvy adults, so it's time to get educated!

The Tire and the Pump: What You Need to Know about His Apparatus

When you're thinking about what a penis is and how it works, picture a tire. Yes, a *tire*, like one of the four on your car wheels.

The inner tube of a tire is like the inner workings of the penis. The rubber skin on the tire is like the penis's skin. You have to fill the inner tube to get a tire to inflate. The tubing of the air pump at the gas station that will fill the inner tube is the equivalent of a man's blood vessels around his penis, and the pump itself is similar to his heart.

That's an important fact to know. When a man becomes

aroused, nerve signals trigger the release of a gas called nitric oxide, which then allows the arteries feeding the penis to open the floodgates and let the blood pump in. A normal erection will last as long as a man is sexually stimulated, or until he reaches orgasm. Then the reverse effect takes place and the blood drains out.

Erections are vital for a penis to stay healthy. When a man is just going about his business, his flaccid penis gets hardly any blood flow. That's a good thing because otherwise he'd be walking around with a permanent hard-on, which wouldn't be good for anyone. But a flaccid penis can't get the oxygen it needs on its own to keep its tissues healthy. The surge of blood during an erection supplies that vital element and also helps remove metabolic waste products that may have collected there.

And you thought his erections were just about sex! Cut your partner some slack when he has erections in his sleep. It's not because he's dreaming of Victoria's Secret models. It's his body doing what it needs to do to keep his penis healthy and functional.

Everything in our body is connected to something else, so problems with a penis aren't necessarily *in* the penis. They can be anywhere. If something is going on with the pump (the heart), such as high blood pressure or heart disease, the penis won't get enough blood and any prospects of sex will go limp, literally. The body needs the pump to pump properly. Gotta have a good heart to have good sex!

You may also be surprised to know that the female anatomy is the same as the male anatomy. The clitoris has the same structure as the penis. It also needs the heart working properly so that blood flow is sufficient for you to have an orgasm. What this means is that men need to have a healthy cardiovascular system for optimal sexual health—and women do, too. (And yes, this means that if you don't get any exercise or need to lose weight, now is the time to start!)

Let's look at some interesting details about the penis.

Dear Dr. Fisch: Morning Glory

Dear Dr. Fisch,

Why does my husband wake up with an erection every morning and want to have sex? I'm too busy trying to get the kids out the door to school and then go to work myself to be in the mood! I'd much rather have sex in the evening, but he's more pooped then. What gives?

Signed, Not in the Mood for Morning Breath (and More)

Dear Not in the Mood for Morning Breath (and More),

You know how your monthly period can make you moody or crave chocolate. The same underlying types of hormonal fluctuations affect all of us every day. For men, testosterone levels tend to peak early in the morning and then drop during the day. (Of course, young men may have fewer dips. Their hormones are in full flush, so they're constantly in the mood, 24/7.)

The reason your husband wakes up so frisky is because he's been having erections all night, what's called nocturnal penile tumescence. As mentioned in the previous section, a man must have these sleep-time erections to get the blood flowing to his penis to keep it healthy. This is basic physiology and absolutely normal, so you don't want this to stop happening or his penis will be in big trouble.

My suggestion would be to work out a schedule where sometimes he gets his morning satisfaction, and sometimes he has to wait for your mood to match his. Good luck!

Yes, You Can "Break" Your Penis (Sort of)

I get asked this all the time. Contrary to the implications of the slang term "boner," the penis doesn't contain a bone—so technically speaking, there's nothing to "break," even though an erection feels fairly hard. However, the outermost layer of the penis (just below the skin) is loaded with ligament-like tissue that can get bent during sex, perhaps during a particularly strenuous session or simply by somebody shifting positions at precisely the wrong moment. This can result in excruciating pain. Doctors refer to the injury as a "fracture" (for expediency, I guess), but it's really a serious strain or tearing of the outermost penile tissue.

If this happens to your guy, get him to a urologist as soon as possible. The penis might seem to heal on its own, but scar tissue can occur, leading to what's called Peyronie's disease. This is a condition in which the penis has a bend or a severe curvature when it's erect. Peyronie's disease can be very painful and make sex very difficult, and it needs medical attention from a urologist because it can't be fixed on its own.

One Size Does Not Fit All

The penis-size topic comes up with such devastating frequency that I wrote a book about men and their penises called *Size Matters:*

The Hard Facts about Male Sexuality That Every Woman Should Know. There is huge variation in penis and testicle size, and men should be reassured to know that even if they worry that they're too small—which nearly all men do, even those who are visibly well-endowed—most are absolutely average in size.

So What's Normal and What's Not?

Men don't usually believe this fact, but bigger is not necessarily better when it comes to an erect penis. A normal adult penis is about three inches long when flaccid and between four and a half and six and a half inches long when erect. The overwhelming majority of men fit into this range, which is good because a penis of that size fits best into the average vagina.

A penis longer than six inches can thrust into a cervix, and that can hurt. But more importantly, only the outer third of a vagina is laden with pleasure-producing nerves, and as you know, your clitoris is outside your vagina. So, even a man with a tiny flute can make a woman very happy if he knows how to play it properly. Since the source of most women's orgasms is the clitoris, your partner may need to directly stimulate you there (and you can help him out).

Trust me, if a man concentrates on foreplay instead of penis insecurities, size will *not* matter. Make that clear to him if your orgasms aren't proof enough! You can also help by telling him how much you love his penis, just the way it is. It's part of him and you adore every bit of him. Repeat this often enough so that he believes you, because this topic can bring out the worst of a man's insecurities.

You might also want to tell him that in a study done in 2005 and reported in the *Journal of Urology*, ninety-two men who'd come to a hospital clinic convinced that they had a "small-sized penis" were evaluated by researchers. Not one of them was actually "small." They were all perfectly average and perfectly normal. The men just thought they were small, and once they were told by researchers to stop worrying, they did!

Does Body Type Have Anything to Do with Penis Size?

Are larger or taller guys naturally more well-endowed? That's another question that I frequently hear. My answer is always the same: A man shouldn't worry about his height correlating to his penis size because that's a myth. All of the scientific studies about penis size I've ever read (and that's been a lot of reading over the years!) found *no* correlation between a guy's height or build and the size of his penis.

In Masters and Johnson's classic studies, the largest penis of the 312 men was about five and a half inches long when flaccid and it was hung on a guy who was 5'7" and weighed 152 pounds. The smallest penis, measuring just two and a half inches when flaccid, was on a guy who was 5'11" and weighed 178 pounds. You'd have thought those statistics would have been reversed!

Dear Dr. Fisch: My Husband Is Still Too Small for Me

Dear Dr. Fisch,
I've been married to my husband, Tony, for two years and love him very much. But his penis is only about three

inches long, even when it's erect. This is really a problem for me because I don't enjoy our lovemaking. And I'm also trying to get pregnant, and this isn't helping. What can we do to make sex better?

Signed, Need a Magnifying Glass

Dear Need a Magnifying Glass,

I can only imagine how difficult this must be for you. Your husband is on the lower side of normal but still considered medically normal. So I suggest you stop thinking about the size of his penis, or lack thereof, and work on having orgasms through other means, since most women do not achieve an orgasm through penile penetration alone.

I'm not saying size doesn't matter, but that there's no reason your husband can't give you plenty of pleasure. You both just need to experiment with different ways to approach foreplay and lovemaking.

Before you get to that point, however, you need to both talk openly about this issue. Yes, it may be embarrassing at first, but, believe me, that's the only way you'll make progress. Having that tough conversation with your husband could be the only way you're going to be able to save your marriage. Like I always say: the answer to any emotional problem is communication, communication, and more communication!

Debunking Bogus Claims (No, He Can't Make His Penis Longer...But He Can Make It Firmer)

I've often seen ads in men's magazines, usually with a handsome, smiling man and lots of exclamation marks, telling men that yes, they can increase their penis size. Sometimes, patients even bring in these ads and look at me hopefully. I hate to tell them the truth. In fact, I can't tell you how many men have fallen for this age-old scam, and it's time we set the record straight. Sadly, no, you *can't* make your penis longer than what your genes and Mother Nature have endowed you with.

Various vacuum devices can produce an artificial erection, but they can't make the penis "bigger." However, they can make a man suffer tremendously because excessive use can leave blood trapped in the penis, leading to gangrene and even death...and that is not the way any man wants to go.

There is also a surgical procedure that can increase the apparent length of the penis by snipping the suspending ligaments. This lets a flaccid penis hang lower, providing an illusion of greater length, but this leads to a floppier penis when erect, so I rarely recommend this be done. Instead, I explain that a man's penis is as unique to him as the shape of his eyebrows or the color of his hair (or, depending on his age, however much hair he still has!).

However, the width of a penis can be increased by increasing the blood flow to it (which is what Viagra and other drugs do)—and this is what women really want. A small penis that is fully engorged tends to be much more satisfying, as most of the sensory nerve fibers in the vagina are found right as you enter the vagina or about an inch inward. A well-rounded penis is going to provide more stimulation there than a long, skinny penis (or what one female friend referred to as a "pencil dick"). The other thing a man can do, of course, is become such a skillful lover—making it clear that he knows that sex is not just about the penis and the vagina—that size is not even thought of as an issue.

Dear Dr. Fisch: What about Equipment Compatibility? Is There Such a Thing?

Dear Dr. Fisch,

Is there such a thing as equipment compatibility, or more like non-compatibility? What I mean is, could there be a penis that just can't fit in a vagina no matter how much chemistry exists out of bed?

Signed, In and Out

Dear In and Out,

Yes, there is such a thing, because of the large range of both penis and vagina sizes. Some fits are simply better than others. If the penis is relatively too big for a small vagina—even if the penis is a perfectly normal size—that's equipment non-compatibility.

This becomes more common as women grow older and develop a condition called atrophic vaginitis. It's caused by a lack of estrogen, making the vagina less elastic and therefore essentially "smaller." This can often be helped with increased use of lubricants. Conversely, some women find that their vaginas become "larger" or more stretched out after childbirth (as famously described in *The Godfather*). This can be fixed by reconstructive surgery called vaginoplasty.

In general, however, most vaginas are very accommodating, especially when women are highly aroused, and most can handle all sizes—but only when lubricated. I can't stress enough that if foreplay is too short and the lubrication is lacking, a vagina will not accommodate a penis of any size without pain. So, foreplay will be your best move for ensuring sexual compatibility with your partner, no matter what equipment you have to play with.

Getting Spunky: The Semen Section

Men don't just worry about size. They can worry about everything having to do with their penis, including what comes out of it. Yes, semen. It can seem fairly innocuous when it's ejaculated, just a small amount of cloudy white fluid. But it is teeming with sperm, so a tiny drop can have a lifetime of consequences for a fertile woman when she is not planning a pregnancy.

In case you were wondering, semen is only about 3 percent sperm. The rest is primarily composed of water, with a mixture of citric acid, amino acids, fructose, enzymes, and a few other minerals. The average volume of a normal ejaculation is between 2 and 5 milliliters, about a teaspoon. (For those of you wondering the age-old question about oral sex and swallowing, semen only has 36 calories!)

Pity the poor sperm, only a few microns long. Its epic journey to the egg of its dreams is a long one because the sperm needs to swim the equivalent of about 100,000 times its own length to get there.

Semen normally tastes fairly sweet and a little bit salty. The fructose in the semen helps power the sperm and keeps them alive on their journey from a man to a woman. But the flavor of semen can be affected by what a man eats or smokes. A bitter taste or pungent smell could be due to smoking (cigarettes or marijuana) or drinking a lot of coffee or alcohol. Some foods, such as asparagus and garlic, can give semen an odd flavor because they contain high levels of certain enzymes or elements. If you consider how your pee smells after you eat asparagus, you know what I mean! Semen might also taste bad if your partner has a low-grade urinary tract infection.

Bottom line: If his semen tastes off or bad and he hasn't been eating anything unusual or smoking or drinking too much, he should get checked out by a doctor to rule out infections or other conditions.

Deal with the "Head": What Affects His Libido?

Now that you know a lot more than you ever thought you'd need to know about penises and sperm, let's move along to how and how often he uses his equipment. In other words, time to talk about his libido.

A man can have trouble with his libido for many physical reasons, and if he is really unlucky (or lazy and self-indulgent) the reason usually falls into one or more of these categories. I've organized this information into an easy-to-remember (and perhaps aptly titled) acronym, HEAD:

H for Hormones

- Hormonal imbalances, congenital conditions (such as small or malformed testicles), erectile dysfunction.

E for Eating (Too Much) and Exercise (Too Much or Not Enough)

- Weight gain (particularly around the waist), sedentary life-style, over-exercising (particularly with weight-training).

A for Aging

- Hormonal changes, prostate issues.

D for Diseases, Drugs, Drinking, and Deprivation (of Sleep)

- Anxiety, depression, osteoporosis, drug use, self-medication, alcohol use, fatigue, sleep disturbances (particularly sleep apnea).

H for Hormones

Testosterone is to men what estrogen and progesterone are to women. It's what separates the men from the women. These are the hormones that drive reproduction and sexual desire.

Along with sperm, testosterone is manufactured in the testicles, and a normal range is anywhere from 300 to 1,100 nanograms per deciliter of blood. The only way to check this level is with a blood test. Be sure to tell your partner to ask for a free testosterone workup. That's not testosterone he gets for free, but what he needs for his body to function properly.

A man with normal testosterone levels tends to have a normal libido. That means he likes sex; he craves sex; and hopefully he has regular, mutually satisfying sex with a partner. A man with low testosterone may have a less intense sex drive and tends to be of the meeker variety (not that this is a bad thing). A man with too much testosterone will make you long for Mr. Meek, because he'll be aggressive, sexually obsessed, competitive, and extroverted—an in-your-face action man.

Unlike women, though, a man shouldn't have fluctuating testosterone levels. His testosterone should remain fairly steady. Still, an estimated two to four million men in America suffer from symptoms associated with below-normal testosterone levels, a condition called hypogonadism. It's very common in men as they grow older, although it can happen to young men, too. Often, it's due to a congenital issue, such as undescended testicles, which don't reach the scrotum, or varicocele, an enlargement of the veins in the scrotum. Both of these issues cause low testosterone levels, often leaving a man too exhausted to have sex and unable to get or sustain erections.

Low testosterone is easy to diagnose with a simple blood test. The most common self-inflicted causes are not getting enough sleep, being overweight, and taking certain medications, such as analgesics like codeine.

The primary symptom of low testosterone is low energy. It's the complaint I hear most frequently. But because so many men are fatigued, they and their doctors often don't think of this hormone as the root cause of the problem. There are simply so many other possible reasons for ongoing exhaustion. These include the stresses of everyday life, a crummy diet (which can lead to prediabetes or diabetes, a disease that wreaks havoc on energy levels), a sedentary lifestyle (lacking regular exercise to give you energy), too much work, and not enough time. Sound familiar? Only about 5 percent of men with hypogonadism are actually being treated for it, leaving millions to suffer.

A healthy adult shouldn't be saying, "I'm getting older so I'm tired." Getting older isn't an automatic recipe for getting pooped. Thinking it is could be a self-fulfilling prophecy, though, or a sign of a much more serious condition. If you have ongoing health issues or changes in how you're feeling, see your physician and get a full blood workup to rule out any problems.

In addition to having fatigue, a man with low testosterone may not be very interested in sex. (I'll discuss medical treatments for erectile dysfunction in "A for Aging," starting on page 106.) Other typical symptoms of low testosterone include muscle weakness, small or soft testicles, erectile dysfunction, sleep disorders, weight gain (particularly around the waist), osteoporosis, depression, anemia, and just plain feeling crummy without knowing why. These are all issues that affect not only a man's health and emotional well-being but yours, too. If your partner doesn't seem to care about sex anymore, the dynamic of your relationship can't help shifting, and this can cause tremendous problems until the root cause is found.

Fortunately, it is much easier for men to raise testosterone levels on their own than for women to raise their estrogen and progesterone without supplements. A man has to be motivated to exercise regularly; eat a nutritious low-carb, low-junk, and low-sugar diet; lose some weight; and quit smoking, drinking, or drugging. With these good habits, a man can naturally improve his testosterone count.

For men who aren't willing to do the work, or whose testosterone levels are severely deficient, hormone replacement therapies can also work wonders. Oral testosterone isn't a feasible option because it is not FDA approved due to an adverse effect on the liver. Gels are by far the most popular application, although injections and patches are also available, all by prescription. Gels are applied daily to the shoulders, upper arms, or abdomen. Used as directed, they usually kick in quickly, bringing a man's testosterone levels back to normal and keeping them there. If low testosterone was the reason for a man's exhaustion and other symptoms, he should be feeling himself again, and his libido should make itself known to you again!

Some men, however, have potentially life-threatening issues affecting them, and lower testosterone is merely a consequence. That's what happened with Phil. He was a big guy, but he'd been a whole lot bigger when I'd first started treating him. I found a pituitary tumor that had been wreaking havoc on his hormones, treated him for it, put him on testosterone, and he lost 150 pounds. He hadn't had sex in *fifteen years*. Once he was in much better physical shape, he wanted to have sex all of the time.

His wife called me up. "I'm not ready for that," she said. She'd gotten used to a sexless relationship. She wasn't sure she even wanted to have sex again. That's not a normal state of mind, so she needed to work with a therapist to address why she was avoiding sex when she could now have it so easily.

They had a lot of work to do to get back to a healthy sexual relationship, believe me!

Low Testosterone and Depression

Another reason it's vital for him to have his testosterone levels checked is that many of the symptoms of low testosterone are similar to those of low-level clinical depression. It's equally as vital to treat the latter as the former to ensure a happy, healthy relationship and sex life for both of you! Any of the following can be symptoms of both:

Low libido
Low energy
Decreased enjoyment of life
Feeing sad or irritable
Sleep disturbances
Problems getting your work done, especially poor
    concentration
Weight gain

Is Testosterone Therapy a Good Thing?

Even though there is a booming business in testosterone replacement therapies, I have a problem with them. As I've said, many men who need testosterone aren't getting it, and many men who don't need it are demanding it. But testosterone replacement therapy is appropriate and safe *only* for men with subnormal levels diagnosed by a doctor or licensed medical professional.

Here's why: certain medical conditions, such as an enlarged prostate or prostate cancer, can be made much worse by testosterone. To say nothing of what it can do to a man's mood and temperament. (Just think of all those angry sports players jacked up on testosterone and steroid shots!) You don't want your usually calm and collected partner morphing into the Hulk because his testosterone has skyrocketed through unnecessary hormone therapy.

In addition, taking testosterone can cause infertility in men. This is great if he doesn't want kids or has them already. It's not great if a couple is trying hard to have a baby. So see a doctor before diving into the deep end of this pool.

E for Eating (Too Much) and Exercise (Too Much or Not Enough)

Eating: Lose the Waist First

As you'll see in the section on Viagra and other pharmaceutical helpers (starting on page 109), erection-enhancing drugs might be thought of as magic pills for erections, but there's no magic pill for weight loss. Actually, there is for me—it's called the Playing Tennis Every Day for an Hour pill. Having an intense workout with a competitive partner keeps me fit and my appetite in check (most of the time). I know I can't stop eating, especially if someone shoves a rib-eye steak or a piece of cheesecake under my nose, so if I didn't exercise, I'd be a blimp!

When I tell my patients that the most common cause of low testosterone is unquestionably excess weight, their eyes widen. They had no idea. I explain that testosterone is broken down in fat cells. Those cells are like greedy little sponges, sopping up all that delectable testosterone gravy and converting it to estrogen-like compounds. If there are a lot of fat cells, the testosterone gravy gets metabolized too quickly, and levels soon drop dangerously low.

You already know that too much fat isn't good for the health of a man's sexual organs or the rest of his body, either. A high-fat and high-sugar diet leads to high cholesterol levels and obesity, which cause an enormous range of health issues—some lethal—and increase the risk of erection problems by lowering testosterone levels. Fat in the blood can clog the small arteries that feed the penis.

Remember, what's bad for the heart is bad for the penis.

I also tell my patients that the goal isn't to lose *weight*; it's to lose the *waist*.

Ideally, waist size for both men and women should be about half your height. I can take one look at a man's belly and have a fairly accurate estimate of his testosterone count—especially bodybuilders weighing 250 pounds of solid muscle. They'll have thirty-two-inch waists despite their weight and are positively teeming with testosterone.

So how much weight is a problem? Based on your own metabolism, think about when you were twenty-one or so. If your weight was normal then, how much do you weigh now? Has there been a significant change? For example, if you were an athlete as a teenager and you weighed 170 pounds, but your weight is now 195, that's too much weight. If your baseline weight was 230 pounds and you're now 240, that might not be as much to worry about.

Healthy bodies come in all shapes and sizes. Consider, for example, Marion Bartoli, who won the ladies' single title at the Wimbledon Championships in 2013. She is shorter and stockier than most other female tennis players, but she is fantastically fit and strong. In my opinion, if your weight is within a normal range, ideally it should remain fairly steady throughout life. (Of course, your physician is the best source of information about appropriate weight for your height and body type.)

I know how hard it is to lose weight. I have men in my office every day who are distraught about their size. If losing weight was easy, no one would be fat. If your partner has a weight problem, my suggestion is that you find a nutritionist who can assess his situation and draw up a realistic eating plan that will fit his lifestyle.

Lose the weight slowly. Cut out the white foods—sugar, rice, potatoes, flour, bread, pasta, baked goods—as much as possible, and add the colorful foods like fruit and veggies and whole grains to your plate. Also, substantial weight loss is nearly impossible unless you add regular exercise to your daily routine.

And have lots more sex—not only does it burn calories, but it is a lot more satisfying than a slab of steak or a bowl of ice cream!

Dear Dr. Fisch: My Belly Fat Won't Budge

Dear Dr. Fisch,

I'm 30, single, and would like to have a better dating and sex life. My problem is that I'm 5'7" and weigh 190 pounds, and most of those pounds are stuck in my belly. I want to lose at least twenty pounds and firm myself up. I try to exercise and I take vitamins, but nothing seems to be working. What am I doing wrong?

Signed, Not a Belly Dancer

Dear Not a Belly Dancer,

First of all, keep your expectations in check. No

one at age thirty should have a six-pack unless he's a professional athlete or model. That's for teenagers. If you're thirty and you have a six-pack, you're working out too much. And you'd rather be dating than doing crunches in the gym, right?

You may have a genetic predisposition for packing the pounds onto your abdominal area. Try working with a trainer for a few sessions to get tips on maximizing your workout to best suit your body. A combination of aerobic exercise and weight training will burn fat and add lean muscle that will raise your metabolism.

A good trainer will also show you exercises that can help firm up your core muscles, which will not only help flatten your belly, but also give you better posture and help prevent lower-back injuries. It's hard to have vigorous sex when your back hurts, right?

Vitamins might be good for your health in general, but they don't contain calories so they can't provide any energy, and they can never help anyone lose weight. (The misperceptions about what vitamins can and cannot do are legion.) The only way to lose weight is with diet and exercise. Are you ready to hear my diet? Drumroll, please. No breads, no pizza, no pasta, no cookies, and no cake.

I know. Sounds horrible, boring, and not what life is all about, but the sugar and starches, or simple carbohydrates, are what's getting to you. They cause your insulin, the hormone that regulates how your body processes sugar, to spike. When this happens, you get hungrier, but any excess calories you'll eat will be stored in your body as fat, particularly in the abdominal area. Ditto with any processed foods, as they're chock full of—you guessed it—sugars and starches.

Look at food as something to help you live a better life—as medicine, almost. Switch to regular (not instant) oatmeal with nuts and some fruit for breakfast. Eat a large salad with some lean meat for lunch, have a steak or roast chicken with lots of veggies for dinner. Just don't eat the potato. That's not so hard, is it? You can have meat and eggs. You can drink milk and eat unsweetened Greek yogurt, and you can eat limitless veggies and more fruit.

If you're going to eat carbs, make them whole-grain only and try brown rice, quinoa, millet, and other unusual grains. They really taste good and they fill you up. Drink water. Lots of water. You are what you eat, of course. Your body will work better when you eat better—improving not just your heart health, but your sexual health, too.

Can you do that? I know you can. Eating crap is a habit. Just think about what you'll look like without that belly. Good sexual health depends on good physical health. Women will flock to you. It's worth it. The food is not.

Sexy Food for a Sexy Him

Yes, a man can eat his way to sexy. High on the list are foods that promote the production of nitric oxide, a necessary gas released in minute amounts to help a penis become erect. Nitric oxide is made from an amino acid called arginine, and to maintain healthy sexual prowess, men should eat foods rich in it, such as:

- Beans
- Walnuts
- Cold-water fish (such as tuna and salmon)
- Soy products
- Oats
- Almonds

Another class of nutrients important for sexual health is bioflavonoids, which are plant compounds that act like antioxidants, those all-important components that scavenge the harmful by-products of the body's metabolism and exposure to environmental pollutants like the sun's radiation, smog, cigarette smoke, or pesticides. Think of them as your body's built-in sanitation department. They increase blood flow to your entire body—and that means your sexual organs, too.

The best sources of bioflavonoids are fruits and vegetables, so everyone should be eating colorful foods every day. Add more color to your food and a lot more spice to your sex life.

Dear Dr. Fisch: I've Hit the Weight Wall— How Do I Break through It?

Dear Dr. Fisch,

I'm 38, 6'4" and I used to weigh more than 400 pounds. I was diagnosed with diabetes, which was finally my wake-up call, and I've managed to lose more than 100 pounds—I'm down to about 285. I exercise regularly but I've hit the wall. No matter how much I work out and what I eat, I can't lose any more weight. It's making me really depressed, and I'm afraid this is going to send me right back to my rotten, old eating habits. What can I do to get back on track?

Signed, Tired of Hitting the Wall

Dear Tired of Hitting the Wall,

Holy smokes! First of all, congratulations on losing those 115 pounds. That's an outstanding accomplishment. What you should do now is see a doctor and get your testosterone checked. Your depression may be related, in part, to low testosterone. Same with your weight-loss plateau. There's no biological reason you can't lose more weight—but you won't be able to do that if you're feeling tired and depressed. If you do have low testosterone, a short-term course of testosterone therapy might kick-start you in a helpful way and give you back your confidence and optimism.

But regardless of your testosterone level, it's important to eat the best food you possibly can and stay away from junk food if that's something you like to indulge in. Ban excess salt and ban sugar. Don't eat anything that's fried. Don't walk into McDonald's if you can help it, or if you do, eat a burger without the bun. Protein is much better for you now than crappy carbs like white bread, pasta, cookies, and other sweets.

And don't think I'm crazy for suggesting this, but a good way for someone who's been dieting for a while and hit the wall to get losing again is to try a vegan diet. This can give you a lot of great, new eating habits and shift the way you think about what you need to put on your plate. Vegan means plants only—fruits, grains, legumes, nuts, and vegetables.

Think of it as a new hobby and start off with one day a week vegan only, then work up to two or three (or more). Do it with your wife and kids, and you'll be shocked at how good you'll feel and how much weight you can lose. And remember—the key to eating lots of salads and veggies is to make a really scrumptious (not sugary or salty) dressing. Even kids who'd rather eat a worm than broccoli will scarf it down if the sauce is outstanding! If you do all these things, you'll be shedding the pounds again in no time. Good luck!

Gaining Weight Can Be a Sexual Problem, Too

Some women and men can eat and eat and eat and never seem to gain any weight. Most of us probably sigh and think, Wouldn't that be a nice problem to have? But it's not, especially not for your sex life.

Gaining much-needed pounds can be as tough for some as losing is for others, especially if they're exercising regularly. But bear in mind that not every man is destined to be two hundred pounds of muscle.

Men who have problems gaining weight may need help from a competent nutritionist, but they should *not* take protein powder to gain muscle mass. Eating lean protein from plant or animal sources is better, because protein powder can cause stomach problems and weight *loss*, the opposite of the desired result. Ideally, you want to be at a normal weight for your height. This makes you less likely to be at risk for weight-related conditions like diabetes, high blood pressure, heart disease, and strokes. And a healthy body is a body that is capable of having satisfying sex on a regular basis.

A man's protein needs will vary with how much he works out. If he works out four to five times a week for an hour or longer, he'll need 55 grams of protein per pound. For a 180-pound man, that translates to about 95 grams of protein per day.

Here's how to gain weight by putting on muscle:

- Eat more! But be sure you're making healthy food choices.
- Eat lean animal- or plant-based protein before and after a workout.
- Stay hydrated by drinking lots of water.
- Eat eggs for their concentrated protein.
- Eat unsweetened yogurt, adding a bit of honey if you need to. Yogurt has an ideal combination of protein and carbs. Greek yogurt has twice the protein of regular yogurt, and is filling and satisfying.
- Drink kefir. This is fermented liquid yogurt that's loaded

with probiotics to help keep the good digestive bacteria in your gut flourishing.

- Eat beef. It's loaded with creatine, which helps muscle growth.
- Eat salmon. This fish is loaded with omega-3 fatty acids, which decrease muscle-protein breakdown.
- Use olive oil, which also decreases muscle breakdown.
- Get enough sleep. All adults need seven to nine hours of sleep a night. LeBron James sleeps about twelve hours a night, and the average athlete sleeps nine to ten hours each night. I have a feeling that's a lot more than you sleep! These athletes know that all of your tissues are replenished at night. Remember, a man's body makes testosterone when he sleeps, so without enough rest, he won't have enough testosterone to give him the energy for a proper workout—especially the kind of workout involving weight training, which demands stamina and power to build muscles. And, of course, the kind of workout he'll want to be having in bed with his partner—namely, you!

Buried Penis Syndrome

When men put on weight, it usually goes to the belly first. I've seen patients who looked fairly normal-sized from the back, but when they turned around, holy cow, their guts practically had lives of their own.

A man whose belly is so large that it obscures his sexual organs has what's called buried penis syndrome. This can make his penis look tiny even if it's of normal size. He might be heartened to know that as soon as he loses the weight, his penis will emerge unscathed and look much larger. That's the best incentive to stop snacking on crap!

Exercise (Too Much or Not Enough)

Everyone needs exercise. A human body is built to move. It is not meant to be sitting at a desk all day—or it will make its displeasure known, and sooner or later (mostly sooner), it's gonna start to ache. It's going to slow down. Muscles will lose their tone and get flabby; internal organs won't function at maximum efficiency because blood flow can become sluggish. Your brain will not get the stimulation and endorphins it craves from regular movement; your energy will lag; and you'll be too pooped to care much about sex.

After all, sex is an athletic event, right? If you or your partner is out of shape, you won't have the stamina for a luscious, long evening of lovemaking. As much as I could inhale the cheesecake I love every day, I'd much rather have great sex than a lot of dessert.

The weight problem is different for men than for women. Men can eat more than women without gaining weight—around 400 calories more each day, basically for three reasons:

- Testosterone. It revs people up, giving them more fat-burning energy. Men have way more of it than you. Not fair, ladies, I know!
- Relative muscle level. Men typically have greater muscle mass per pound than women. Muscle tissue naturally weighs

more than fat tissue, and the more a man has, the more he'll raise his metabolism because muscle cells burn calories faster than other types of cells. This is one of the reasons why women need to do weight training—not only does it strengthen your muscles, but by adding muscle mass, you will also increase your metabolism.

- His genes and your genes. Just as a man has no control over how tall he's going to be, or how soon he's going to lose all the hair he desperately wants to keep, he has no control over whether he can eat like a pig and stay slim, due to genetic factors making his stomach a furnace, or be like most of the rest of us who have to watch what we eat and work out all the time. Walk down any busy street, and you'll certainly see as many overweight men as overweight women.

Let's get back to testosterone levels. A man who is in good shape due to regular aerobic and weight-training exercise is a lot more likely to have a higher libido than a man who sits at his desk all day and doesn't find the time to work out. A man's body must have adequate testosterone levels to build muscle mass, so someone who is fit and muscled is likely to have normal or high levels of testosterone. (As you already know, low testosterone can make it difficult for a man to have or maintain his erections.) However, an adult man who struggles to gain weight or put on muscle despite regular workouts must get his testosterone checked, pronto.

Bottom line: Just as you know you need to incorporate exercise into your daily life, so do men. If they're sedentary, they should start slowly and not go crazy on the weight machines or free weights because they *will* get hurt. And if your man starts lifting weights obsessively, he might find it hard to lose weight, because adding all that muscle quickly makes a man insatiably hungry. The best thing to do is find a resistance-training program that gradually increases muscle mass. This will keep his appetite in check and help get the weight off.

You might also suggest that you work out together. If you can both join a gym and coordinate your schedules, that is a fantastic incentive. You don't have to do the same workout, but you'll be less likely to cancel if you're committed to meeting at a certain time. Or, see if he can join a team. He might not get quite as much exercise on a team as if he went for long runs, but the camaraderie is a ton of fun, and whenever exercise is fun, it's a lot less likely to fall off the calendar.

Bear in mind, too, that when a sedentary, overweight man starts exercising, he might gain a small amount of weight at first from the muscle mass he's adding to his body. This should be followed by a significant weight loss once the new muscles increase his metabolic rate.

To lose weight smartly, men (and anyone for that matter) should walk a minimum of 10,000 steps each day. That will improve his heart health and gradually increase his stamina. If there's a question of how many steps your guy is walking, get him a pedometer, which tracks the number of steps. If he doesn't get close to that number, try to have him walk around the neighborhood for a while (if at all possible) or do a DVD or streaming workout until he does.

Whatever workout he chooses, it should be something he likes so he'll stick to it. I see men in the gym every day, running on the treadmills and bored out of their minds. They're not working out at maximum capacity because they don't really enjoy it. I can exercise as much as I do because tennis is one of my great passions and stress relievers. That keeps me on the courts even when I've had an exhausting day. It keeps me fit and strong, and it keeps my libido juicy.

A for Aging

A common question my older patients ask me is: When do you become a sexual senior?

My answer: When you feel like one!

I've lost count of how many sixty-something male patients have sat in my office worrying about their age and their cholesterol and minor aches and pains.

"Do you have morning erections?" I ask them.

They nod yes.

"Do you have regular sex, at least two to four times a week?"

They nod yes.

"Then you're healthy."

They look at me in shock.

"The penis is the dipstick of a man's health," I explain. "A well-functioning penis and a regular sex life mean your body is working as it should. Of course you should still have regular medical checkups, but this is one of the best indicators a man can have that he's in good shape."

They nod again, smiling happily.

"If, on the other hand, your sexual drive starts to decline," I hasten to add, "and if you only feel like having sex once or twice a month, or once or twice a year, that tells me something's wrong, and it needs to be investigated. But in the meantime, enjoy yourself!"

The Male Biological Clock, or Why the Lucky Guy Doesn't Get Hot Flashes

When it comes to aging, women have it rough. Not only do you go through hormonal hell every month while you are fertile, but you can go through an even worse hormonal hell during perimenopause, when the female hormones estrogen and progesterone start to decline, and during menopause, when these hormones decline even more rapidly.

Men don't age in quite the same way. While women can find their hormonal drops to be rather precipitous, testosterone levels gradually slide down the slope by only about 1 percent each year, usually starting around the age of thirty. As a result, a man's chronological age is not the best kind of indicator of where his biological clock stands.

I know men in their seventies and, rarely, in their eighties who have the sexual stamina of a man fifty years their junior. Now that's saying something. Conversely, a man in his thirties with low testosterone will have the sexual stamina of his grandfather. For him, that's saying something, too — only not in the way he wants!

The best way to gauge the male biological clock is by measuring three physical factors:

- Testosterone (how high the level)
- Erections (the quality and reliability)
- Weight gain (within a normal range, especially waist size)

A man who's not having any difficulties with these three factors is considered biologically young even if he is chronologically old, although the quality of the genetic material in sperm does degenerate with age.

Still, as both men and women grow older, both take longer to become aroused. Women have less vaginal lubrication, and men's erections aren't as high or as robust (what I already called the angle of the dangle). And lots of other factors come into play, because overall health also determines sexual health and sexual aging. These factors include how well a man takes care of himself by: eating nutritious food and exercising regularly, getting enough sleep, not smoking, avoiding excessive alcohol or drug consumption, not having other illnesses or accidents, and avoiding exposure to environmental hazards, as well as by the luck of the draw with his genetic history. Obviously, women need to deal with these same factors, as well as the physical changes that come with large drops in hormonal activity over the perimenopause years.

Eventually, of course, men need to confront their mortality the way you women often already do. I know how my wife felt when she realized her fertile years were behind her. Although we already had three teenage children by then, for her as for so many other women, it was still is a shock to realize that she was getting older and there's no turning back that clock. A man coming to grips with his aging penis will be struggling with the same feelings.

Older couples who come to see me frequently ask what the secrets are to keeping up a gratifying sex life as they start to slow down. I'll address this more in Part II, but overall, the key for both men and women is to keep your relationship strong through a few basics that you may have already heard. Foster great communication with your partner; help each other feel secure and loved; keep desire alive with a willingness to experiment and try new things;

and adapt playfully to the bodily changes that accompany aging. You have to do your best to laugh about getting older, because, as the old cliché goes, the alternative could be worse.

And, of course, there's the miracle of modern medicine for men—in the form of the little pills that have revolutionized the treatment of sexual dysfunction, and can ease the stresses and strains and worries about aging because they keep those erections coming. (Sorry, bad pun!)

The Infamous "Vitamin V": Viagra and Other Pharmaceutical Helpers

Lots of my patients jokingly refer to their little blue Viagra pills as their own special "Vitamin V."

Viagra made a huge splash when former presidential candidate Bob Dole did commercials for it on TV after its initial launch in 1998. Pundits were incredulous—here was a politician, a statesman, a public figure, no less, speaking candidly and without shame about a man's need for a sexual aid because the natural effects of age had slowed him down. Talk about courage!

The point of Bob Dole's story is that no man with sexual dysfunction, no matter what his age, should be embarrassed about needing medical help to improve the quality, duration, and frequency of his erections. As I've said already, it is perfectly normal for men to have some kind of sexual dysfunction at some point in life—usually from a temporary situation like stress or fatigue or the emotional anxiety of having a new sexual partner. A decrease in sexual prowess is also to be expected as years go by. Blame it on biology and the fact that we age and slow down.

That said, if a man is having any problem with a loving partner

in bed, he should make an appointment with his doctor or a urologist to discuss it and options for treatment (both medical and
non-medical). Once medical reasons such as low testosterone or
other factors are ruled out, and when warranted and truly needed,
erection-enhancing drugs (EEDs) like Viagra, Levitra, and Cialis
can be just the kind of oomph a guy needs. Sometimes just knowing that there are meds to help with erections is all a man needs to
get over whatever is keeping him down.

And it's not only about his needs. Your needs are just as important. A man who knows that he can easily get a little oomph to
help him perform is a man who will regain his sexual confidence.
That should make you both happy, in bed and out.

Although testosterone declines very slowly over the years, a
man of fifty will still have about 20 percent less testosterone than
he did when he was thirty. With those numbers, and factoring in
other conditions such as weight, diet, cardiovascular health, and
different medical conditions, it's been estimated that 50 percent
of men between the ages of fifty and sixty have some level of
erectile dysfunction. Sixty percent of men at age seventy do, as do
70 percent of those at age eighty or above. For them, EEDs can
be fantastic.

EEDs work by blocking an enzyme that controls the way arteries in the penis constrict after the release of nitric oxide, making it
easier for a man to get an erection and to maintain it. It's important to note that EEDs do not *cause* erections. Nitric oxide needs
to already be present in the penis—and as you read on page 78,
nitric oxide is only produced by your body in response to physical or mental sexual stimulation. This is a good thing, because
otherwise every man taking an EED would walk around with an

erection for hours, if not days, and that can be a *huge* impediment to normal functioning.

In a man who doesn't need that extra boost, an EED will enhance his erection by adding a maximal amount of blood into the penis. Because he'll have a shorter latency period, he might be able to have another erection in less time. He can ejaculate again, too. This can be a good thing for you if he was too quick for you to be able to have an orgasm the first time. A second erection can slow him down and give you the time you need for your own pleasure.

But if the desire for sex isn't there, an EED is not going to work. EEDs also don't work well in men with low testosterone and the ensuing low libido. But if hormone replacement therapy works, the EEDs should, too. Viagra and Levitra need to be taken about thirty to sixty minutes before sexual activity is expected. The effects typically last for four to six hours. Cialis got its nickname as "the weekender" because its effects stick around for about thirty-six hours, which gives a man a larger window for the time when he wants to have sex.

If the EEDs don't work and testosterone levels are normal, further medical intervention may be required. There might be some other medical issue, or perhaps damage to either the blood vessels or nerves involved with erections. There are erection-creating options such as self-injection into the penis, intra-urethral suppositories (yes, just what it sounds like!), vacuum devices, and penile implants, but all have their drawbacks and are treatments of last resort.

The Overuse of Erection-Enhancing Drugs

As a urologist who has seen the emotional pain, worries, and suffering that men robbed of their ability to have satisfying and regular sex suffer from, you might think I'd be brimming with joy that EEDs are so widely prescribed, used, and accepted. After all, before these pills were created, many men were unable to have a healthy and happy sex life due to erectile dysfunction. Now that these pills can alleviate some of this dysfunction, it should be a win-win for these men and their partners, right?

Not so fast. Yes, EEDs can be near-miracle workers for men who really need them. But because EEDs are all too often dispensed the way antibiotics are—for illnesses that don't really require them—and scarfed down by men who don't have a clue about the real cause of their erectile dysfunction, EEDs fall into the category of overprescribed and overused.

Since erectile dysfunction can be an early sign of a serious medical problem, a prescription for an EED should *never* be dispensed unless a man's overall health is properly assessed first. Conditions like diabetes, heart disease, or cancer that may be causing the erectile problems need to be ruled out.

Lots of men don't want to know this, so they doctor-shop until they get the prescription they want. (Please do not get me started on medical practitioners who prescribe improperly!) For these men, having erections when they want them is more important than taking optimal care of their health. Lots of younger guys take EEDs to reduce performance anxiety, too.

Remember, any man willing to potentially risk his well-being simply to have more sex is taking chances with his health. Make it clear to him that pill-popping is never a substitute for common sense and self-worth.

Dear Dr. Fisch: Pill-Popping Peter

Dear Dr. Fisch,

My husband, Peter, can't have sex without popping a little blue pill. It makes me feel like I can't satisfy him on my own. Am I wrong to think that way?

Signed, Feel Like a Drug Dealer When I'm Not

Dear Feel Like a Drug Dealer When I'm Not,

I used to joke that if a man's wife has a problem with him taking Viagra, then he's with the wrong woman, because as long as he's able to have an erection and satisfy both his partner and himself, that's all that matters. But that's only a joke!

In truth, you raise a valid concern. I understand your worries because I agree completely with how you feel. Popping a pill instead of candidly discussing his fears of sexual dysfunction is not a great way for your husband to have a vibrant sexual or emotional relationship.

If Peter has seen a urologist who did a thorough examination and concluded, based on blood work, that Peter really needs Viagra, then the pill is a necessity for his erections to happen. If, on the other hand, Peter never saw a urologist or other medical professional who measured his testosterone levels, he should see a doctor or find a better doctor who will thoroughly evaluate him to make sure the pills are really needed.

Most of all, tell him how you feel. You also can change your foreplay, doing things to your husband that you know he finds sexually stimulating, so that you'll feel like a more active participant early on.

Don't Buy Prescription Meds for Sexual Dysfunction over the Internet!

This may seem like a no-brainer, but you wouldn't believe how many people do this. First of all, it's illegal to sell prescribed medications to Americans over the Internet without a prescription. Just because websites and spam emails advertise these drugs, many of which are controlled substances, doesn't mean these sites are legitimate.

Aside from encouraging buyers to self-medicate, which can cause further medical issues or even be lethal, the biggest problem with these websites is that the buyer has zero ability to verify if these drugs have been manufactured properly or are the real things. Many come from countries like India, where regulations in the drug-manufacturing industry are minimal at best and, in many cases, nonexistent.

Drug manufacturers looking to cut corners might make pills that are not much more than placebos, with little if any of the active compounds you're looking for. Or you could get something laced with arsenic, concrete, or other harmful substances due to a deliberate lack of manufacturing quality control. Not only that, but these sites will then have your credit-card information and can sell it to the unscrupulous. You could end up with a bad erection, along with a bad case of identity theft.

It's never worth risking your physical and financial health to get prescriptive drugs or treatments through these sites. Find a doctor you like and trust, and be aware that what you don't know about your meds can not only kill your sex life—it can kill *you*.

Dear Dr. Fisch: I Think My Husband Is Addicted to Viagra!

Dear Dr. Fisch,

I'm sixty, and my husband is sixty-two. He takes Viagra so he can keep it up during sex. But I'm worried that he's scarfing down too many and maybe should stick with a pill that only needs to be taken a couple times a week, versus one that has to be taken daily. What kinds of erection-enhancing meds should he use?

Signed, Pill-Counting Wifey

Dear Pill-Counting Wifey,

Let me congratulate you before I say anything else, because if you're still having an active sex life at your age, you're doing great! Having sex several times a week is a very good sign for both you and your husband and the health of your relationship.

But I understand your concerns, so let me explain the difference between a pill like Viagra, that your husband would take only when he wants to have sex (and no more than once a day), and the pills he is able to take less often. All three erection-enhancing drugs work well. Viagra and Levitra each last for about four hours. Cialis can be taken the same way that he'd take Viagra, but its effect lasts up to thirty-six hours. Your husband needs to discuss his options with his urologist.

Your husband might prefer taking a daily pill. Cialis is available that way at a dosage of five milligrams per day. This may be what your husband is taking. Many older men find that this daily dose helps preserve the spontaneity because they don't have to think about whether they've taken the pill when they're feeling frisky. A lot of them also find that a daily pill helps them urinate better. The decision really comes down to personal preference.

Whatever you both decide, as long as your husband is otherwise in good health—his weight is normal, he doesn't smoke, he doesn't drink a lot, and he eats well—you two sound quite admirable to me. Maintaining a quality sex life at your age will keep you happy with each other and guarantee you many more years of enjoyment and pleasure together.

D Is for Diseases, Drugs, Drinking, and Deprivation (of Sleep)

In this section, I'm going to discuss the D topics—you know, the problems that often happen when you live in denial about your health. I've seen umpteen patients over the years who are smart, successful, loving, generous men but who just don't want to know what's going on with their bodies. Often that doesn't change until I tell them that a man who has health issues is not a man who wants to have sex—or is capable of having great sex!—and that it's time to get serious about their bodies.

D for Diseases

Getting a man to the doctor for his five-point checkup (see the box "Basic Blood Tests Every Man Needs") is not always an easy task. Women tend to be much more attuned to their bodies, and I think that because they see their gynecologists for regular check-ups, they have a better gauge of their overall health. Men, on the other hand, can be stubborn creatures who take body denial to a whole new level, one so high that they can put themselves at grave risk of becoming seriously ill or even dying.

Recently, I heard about a Princeton PhD who had an extremely high PSA (prostate-specific antigen) number but dismissed it because false positives are common with that test. When he collapsed over a year later, he underwent several months of intrusive and painful testing only to discover that he had Stage IV prostate cancer, the most advanced level. Had he (and his doctor) used common sense and repeated the original PSA test just in case, he might have discovered the cancer before it metastasized and went into his bones.

Basic Blood Tests Every Man Needs

When men come to me for treatment, I always recommend a full blood workup, because it's extremely important that all men have their "five numbers" assessed. These are:

Glucose level (to check for diabetes)
Blood pressure (to check his circulation)

Cholesterol (to check his heart health)

PSA (to check the prostate-specific antigen and his prostate health)

Testosterone (to check his sex hormone levels)

Just Because You Can Buy It Doesn't Mean It's Good for You!

Before starting any course of medications, a man should always ask his doctor what these meds can do to his libido.

While many drugs prescribed for non-sex-related medical issues are necessary for health reasons, they can be extremely detrimental to a man's sexual health and fertility. Certain painkillers, like those containing codeine, can lower testosterone levels, for example. Drugs prescribed to control urinary flow affect ejaculation. Meds that should be avoided overall, such as anabolic steroids, cause shrinkage of the testicles. Antidepressants are notorious for lowering libido in men and women.

If drugs like these need to be prescribed, the man (or woman) should have a candid discussion with his doctor or therapist about the severity of his condition, how long he might need to be on the medication, and what he should do if his libido is affected but his partner's isn't.

Options for switching the medication should be discussed, too. Some medications are easier to switch than others, depending on your condition and potential side effects. It's a constant balancing act between needing to take care of specific issues and being aware that other aspects of your life might be affected for the short term. I've found that a lot of patients find it much easier to deal with a potential lessening of libido if they are told that it's only for a few months, rather than for years, and that they should concentrate on dealing with one medical condition at a time.

Furthermore, people often don't realize that over-the-counter drugs can have the same inhibiting effects on sexual health as certain prescription medications. This goes for some of most innocuous meds that many people take on a regular basis. For example, Sudafed or similar medications like Claritin D with pseudoephedrine can also cause erection problems by not allowing the blood flow to get into the penis. These drugs work by decreasing the blood vessels in your nose, which means they have an effect on blood vessels found elsewhere in the body (like the penis). Prescription pain relievers that are narcotic analgesics, like codeine, can cause pituitary suppression in men, which causes their testosterone levels to drop like stones thrown into a pond.

You already know that I seriously discourage self-diagnosis. This is why good doctors always ask their patients for a comprehensive list of all the meds they're taking, including vitamins—so don't be embarrassed if you take OTC meds or herbal supplements. Don't forget to list everything, including any OTC meds you swallow regularly, such as aspirin or allergy medicines. You certainly don't want to be misdiagnosed as having a serious medical condition or sexual dysfunction caused by an illness when the actual cause is triggered by your OTC meds.

D for Drugs and Drinking

This section is short but not so sweet, because if a man abuses drugs or alcohol, he's eventually going to have serious problems in bed. Not just because he's passing out or too high or plastered to take care of himself (or you!), but because these substances depress the central nervous system. This can disrupt the proper flow of blood to the penis, leaving a man unable to have or maintain an erection. Ditto with smoking because it also constricts blood vessels (and who wants to kiss a chimney?). That means he may get aroused but he won't be able to be a satisfactory lover.

In addition, drugs like marijuana or cocaine, or even a few cocktails, lower inhibitions. They affect the pleasure centers in your brain. Consequently, harder drugs like heroin or other opiates usually make erections practically impossible.

If your partner's in the mood yet feels that he can't have sex without a prop in the form of a few drinks, a few pills, or a few smokes or snorts, then something is wrong. You need to talk, and he needs to be sure he's eating good food, getting good exercise, managing his stress as best he can, and getting enough sleep. If the problem persists, he should probably get professional help from his doctor or a therapist.

You don't need me to go into all the reasons why excessive drugging and drinking are bad for anyone's overall health, mentally and physically. As with other health issues previously discussed, it's not just your sex life you save—it's your life, period.

Do Aphrodisiacs Actually Work?

Aphrodisiacs have been written about—and ingested— for centuries in nearly every culture. They have nearly caused the extinction of the rhinoceros (for its horn), the tiger (for its penis), and the shark (for its fin), all of which supposedly can enhance people's attractiveness and libido.

They have inspired the endless consumption of oysters, herbs, powders, potions, ointments, liniments, creams, elixirs, and even the crushed shells of rather nasty-looking beetles (otherwise known as "Spanish fly," even though they weren't Spanish and they weren't flies). Did any of them work? No, they did not. Not physically at least.

But if someone believes strongly enough in the placebo effect—where he is positive that ingesting some substance, no matter how inert, will work in the way he wants it to—chances are high that the bogus crap he swallowed might just "work" after all. Believe me, the placebo effect is real and has been extensively documented in controlled scientific studies.

I say, as long as the substance isn't harmful to you, your partner, or the environment (no more rhino horns, please), feel free to try these—within reason. More power to any brain that believes what it wants to believe and the body that follows its command if it ends up making you feel good!

Modern aphrodisiacs, on the other hand, aren't just placebos. Some of them are drugs, and when you take them, your body is going to react. The most notorious of these are "poppers," or alkyl nitrites, which have been around for more than fifty years and can enhance sexual response. And as I've said, stimulant drugs like cocaine and methamphetamines may turn a man on, but they often cause erectile dysfunction at the same time. So can opiates like heroin or opium. So can alcohol. So can marijuana. So can prescription painkillers. The problem is that these drugs all inhibit the body's ability to follow through on that urge. In other words, the mind might be willing but the body is too drugged to cooperate!

High doses of testosterone might also increase sexual desire, but they can cause infertility and other side effects, such as aggression, shrinking of the testicles, acne, and urination problems. All in all, there's no substitute for a real sexual connection with a partner!

D for Deprivation (of Sleep)

The number one reason why people are tired is that they don't get enough sleep. The average man or woman needs seven to nine hours of sleep a night, according to the National Sleep Foundation (NSF). Do you get that much? Judging from the flurry of sleep studies and media surrounding sleeping issues, I bet you don't.

In fact, the NSF reported that between 1959 and 1992, the average amount of sleep decreased from eight to nine hours per night to seven to eight hours, and those numbers continue to decline. We're stressed, we're worried about the economy and taking care of our families, and we can't turn off those electronic devices that keep our minds too engaged to drift off to the Land of Nod.

When you're exhausted, usually the last thing on your mind is sex. Sex requires mental and physical energy, and all you want is the sweet oblivion of deep, restful, blessed sleep...where your guy won't disturb you with his morning erections, the baby won't be screaming, and your boss won't call at 6:00 a.m. to remind you that you promised to cover for a colleague who is a notorious slacker.

Lack of sleep is not just something to joke about, though. It is devastating. People who are tired are less productive. Their reflexes are off. They are more prone to accidents and mistakes. Kids don't do as well in school. Parents mess up at work. And, of course, when you're exhausted, it's harder to manage everything. Like your temper. I can't tell you how many patients have told me about fights at home, all triggered because someone was ready to collapse from sleep deprivation and just snapped.

So what does this have to do with a man's sex drive? First of all, testosterone is manufactured during the deepest levels of sleep. Without it, a man's libido can plummet. He not only won't want to have sex but also will have a difficult time achieving an erection.

Sometimes men are sleep deprived because they're getting up several times during the night to use the bathroom. This increased nighttime urination might be a sign of prostate problems. But I'm usually more worried about their sleeping patterns than their prostate. My hunch is that many overly tired men are suffering from sleep apnea.

This isn't snoring, which can happen to anyone. Sleep apnea is a condition where you literally stop breathing when you're sleeping, then wake up gasping for air. Not only can you asphyxiate yourself (in rare cases), but sleep apnea can also be responsible for higher instances of heart disease, stroke, and diabetes. And because it leaves sufferers exhausted from chronically interrupted sleep, they won't be thinking about sex or pleasuring their partners. They'll just be desperate to conk out.

Why do so many men have sleep apnea? During sleep, air is drawn in through your mouth and passes by your uvula, a fleshy part of your throat near your tonsils. As men get older and often put on weight, the tissue around the uvula thickens, making it more difficult for a clear flow of air to get down to the lungs. Men with sleep apnea start snorting and making choking noises and their hearts race. They wake up with a startle, and then they go back to sleep and the cycle starts all over again.

This is unbelievably disruptive—not just to them, but to anyone sleeping in the bed with them. Your own sleep can be so disturbed, leaving you exhausted and worried about your partner's breathing, that it can seriously harm your relationship. I know that when I don't get enough sleep, I am crabby, cranky, and crummy to be around. Sleep deprivation leaves you on edge and ready to pick a fight when you don't mean to.

While sleep apnea doesn't go away on its own, men can help alleviate some of the symptoms by losing weight, if it needs to be lost, and no longer smoking and drinking, both of which can exacerbate the condition considerably

If your partner is chronically exhausted, and if you or he notices the signs of sleep apnea, he must see his doctor and discuss his options. Often, a night in a sleep lab can provide the data needed so treatment can be prescribed. Typically, a CPAP (continuous positive airway pressure) machine is set up for him to use at night. This is a mask attached to a small box that increases air pressure in the throat so the airway stays open without collapse when he breathes in. It's not exactly the sexiest thing you'll want him wearing, but what do looks matter when it might save his life and your sex life?

Dear Dr. Fisch: Is My Sleep Apnea Killing My Libido?

Dear Dr. Fisch,

I just found out that I've got really low testosterone (down to 109). My doctor said I have sleep apnea and I've been using the CPAP box, but I still feel crummy and sex is a distant memory. What else can I do?

Signed, CPAP Really Is CRAP

Dear CPAP Really Is CRAP,

Your testosterone level is really low. Women, on average, have a level of about thirty, and the average for men is more like six hundred. Yours shouldn't be any lower than three hundred. Something's going on, and as annoying as it may be, I'm glad you've got the CPAP device. That will definitely help your sleep apnea and raise your nightly production of testosterone.

If you're carrying around any extra weight or belly fat, you should also take steps to lose that. Especially around the torso, fat acts like a testosterone sponge, sucking that hormone out of your blood, where it should be, and storing it in fat cells.

But your testosterone level is so low that I suspect something else may be going on. I recommend getting a blood test for prolactin and thyroid function, in addition to having your testosterone test repeated. If your prolactin level is elevated, you might have a benign pituitary tumor that's causing your hormone levels to get out of whack.

If so, the treatment is to use medication to shrink the tumor. If that doesn't work or the tumor is severe, then surgery is warranted. It's important to test thyroid function as well because low levels of your thyroid hormones, which regulate your metabolism, can also make you feel sluggish and lacking in energy. Make sure your doctor does these tests, and you should get answers soon.

About Infertility

Another health issue that can have devastating effects on male libido is infertility.

Infertility is a devastating condition for any couple trying to get pregnant. It is, unfortunately, also incredibly common. More than 2.5 million American men are unable to father a child the regular way through sexual intercourse. Because the infertility issue is often assumed to lie with the woman when she is unable to conceive, many couples suffer needlessly for years without bothering to test the man's fertility thoroughly (or perhaps at all). In reality, men and women are equal. Roughly 40 percent of infertility is caused by the woman and 40 percent is caused by the man. In the remaining 20 percent, either both partners contribute or the cause is unknown.

There are many reasons for male infertility, including:

- Problems with the number, shape, or motility (swimming ability) of sperm
- Ejaculation problems
- Congenital lack of sperm
- Congenital malformations of the reproductive tract
- Infections of the reproductive tract
- Sexually transmitted diseases
- Hormonal abnormalities

One extremely important point for child-bearing couples: If a man is taking testosterone supplements, this can reduce or eliminate his fertility. He'll have to stop the supplements and boost his levels naturally by eating right, getting enough sleep, and exercising regularly.

The only way to deal with infertility is by seeing a specialist and going through a battery of tests. Don't despair! There are many options to be explored and it is possible to father a child even with an extremely low sperm count.

Can You Tell from Just Looking That a Man Is Fertile?

Just as men are biologically programmed to want sex in order to perpetuate our species, women are also biologically programmed to look for a man who is fertile enough to get her pregnant so she can contribute to this species perpetuation in her own way. So how do you know if a man is good in bed? If he's in good shape and he looks healthy. Why is that?

A man who is fit and trim is *much* more likely to be fertile than a man with a large belly. One of the biggest turnoffs to a woman, whether she realizes it or not, is a man with a large belly. She might just think it doesn't look attractive and would be difficult to navigate if not downright painful during sex, but the reality is that the larger a man's waist, the lower his testosterone level, since you need normal testosterone levels to make sperm. So a man with a large gut is going to be less fertile and subliminally (as well as visibly) less attractive.

Another way to tell if a man is fertile can't be seen when a guy is dressed, but once he's naked, you can make a rough guess by the size of his testicles. There is as much variation in the family jewels as there is in penis size, but on average, a normal testis is about the size of a walnut in the shell, or about one-and-a-half to two inches in length. Too small (the size of cherries) usually means that he may have a low sex drive due to low testosterone.

Since 95 percent of a testicle is sperm-producing cells, and the remaining 5 percent produces testosterone cells, a small testicle makes a smaller amount of sperm and testosterone. Or, if he is taking testosterone replacements, his levels will soar into the stratosphere while his balls themselves will shrink into tiny nubs. (Not sexy in the slightest, right?) Too big means he might have a collection of fluid or a lot of veins that make him believe the testicle is large when it isn't. (This must be treated by a urologist.) Too hard also means that he needs to see a urologist to rule out any maladies. Too walnut-y means just right!

LESSON 4

RISKY BUSINESS
PORNOGRAPHY, AFFAIRS, AND SEXUAL ADDICTION

Sure, sex is great. It's wonderful. If done right with the right person, it makes you feel better than you've ever felt before. But sex is risky, no matter who you are.

Any time you take your clothes off with another person, it's risky behavior. Even if it's the person you married and have been having sex with for twenty years. So I'm going to tackle the tough stuff that comes along with risks—pornography, affairs, and sexual addiction.

You know by now that some of the best things in life come to those who take risks—going far from home to college, perhaps, or accepting a job in a start-up company; falling in love or raising children—but those are the good kind of risks. The kind that you're willing to take because you've thought them through, and you're willing to accept the consequences of whatever might happen, good or bad.

Sex, on the other hand, isn't about thinking it through. It's about living in the moment. And while that can be a mind-blowing, amazing moment, it can also become a very dangerous moment very quickly.

That's because once you start having sex, you are focused on only one thing. *Having sex.* Your normal, rational, smart, and responsible brain function stops. Your inhibitions disappear. All the precautions you'd normally take—like the condoms in the drawer next to your bed so you can be assured of safe sex—are forgotten. Can't get to those condoms in time? Oh, don't worry; you don't need them. Not when it feels so good and so right and you…just…can't…stop! Why, it's *impossible* to stop.

Nothing will happen, right?

Sure it won't. Repercussions only happen to other people, right? Until they happen to *you.*

That's why about 50 percent of all pregnancies in this country are unintentional. Talk about life changing. Talk about scary.

And they aren't the only thing that's scary or risky. There are STDs. There are betrayals. There are ruined marriages and devastated children. There are lost jobs and ruined reputations when employees get caught downloading or watching porn at work. And there are public humiliations when cheating or sexting is exposed.

That said, sex doesn't *have* to be as risky as it is when you throw all caution to the wind with yourselves on the bed. Once you know that your brain is going to check out when you need it the most, you can train it to outwit your libido and still have lots of great sex. You can prepare.

All you have to do is think of sex as a sport, like tennis or football, and think of yourself as an athlete in training.

After all, how do professional athletes train? They put in countless hours of practice, not just to make their muscles strong but to create what's called "muscle memory." When your muscle memory is honed, you know it's there. You can call on it without thinking. That's why even the world's best ballet dancers go to class every day. They're repeating the basic steps they've done literally millions of times already, but they're perpetuating good habits. Once they do that, they can perform flawlessly and safely without even thinking about it.

Ditto with playing tennis or football once you're on the court or playing field. What happens during the game might not be exactly what you did in practice, but you'll still be primed to plan for contingencies and backup plans, should everything go south. The game will always move too fast for you to be able to stop and analyze every moment, but your reflexes will have been primed.

In other words, if you've prepared enough, your muscle memory takes over and you play safely and to the best of your abilities.

The whole point of all this preparation is not just to play a killer game, but to be able to anticipate any potential winning or losing situations before they happen—so you can score the way you want to. So *you* can be in control.

Same with sex. The more you prepare, the lower your risk. For example:

- If you practice smart sex habits, you will always have the condoms on hand, so you won't have to fumble for them or not bother using them in the heat of the moment.
- If you're not in a committed relationship, you'll have already said, "You need to put this on" so many times that you'll have no problem saying it again or your partner will automatically reach for them. Your mantra is "No glove, no love," and you stick to it!
- You'll take your birth control pills without fail or be vigilant

about other effective forms of birth control so you won't
have to worry about getting pregnant.

- You'll research the pros and cons of anal sex and insist on
proper precautions before you allow it to happen.
- You'll get the HPV vaccine to lower your risk of catching
the virus.
- You'll make it clear that no means no if your partner wants
to experiment with some form of sexual behavior you're
not comfortable with.

Then you'll let your muscle memory take over, and you'll have
a fantastic, orgasmic time in bed because you won't have to worry
about the risks, and you can just concentrate on the pleasure of
the moment that you deserve!

Porn Is Killing Sex in America (No, I Am Not Exaggerating!)

Speaking of pleasure, and there is, of course, much to be had in
bed, one of the biggest pleasure-killers available is streaming 24/7
into bedrooms across America and the rest of the world. You
already know I'm talking about—pornography.

The porn industry seems to be making a shocking amount of
money. Never before has so much sexually explicit imagery been
so easily and inexpensively available. What transformed porn from
something difficult to see (slinking into Times Square back when
it was seedy, or ordering "blue" movies to surreptitiously screen
on the home projector in the basement) to practically mainstream
was home video.

As soon as the format was invented and VCRs became popular,

so did porn—even more so when videos were supplanted by easier-to-use DVDs. And then there was the proliferation of cable channels, which often hosted late-night raunch, and the appearance of pay-per-view porn selections in hotel rooms. Now, of course, more free pornography is out there streaming 24/7 on the Internet than any man could watch in a lifetime.

I sometimes think that the ground-zero moment for the obesity epidemic was the invention of the microwave oven. It made "cooking" ultra-easy and eating far too easy. A whole new category of junk food was created, and all you had to do was hit a button and wait a minute or two before you could eat it. In the same way, the ground-zero moment for porn, in my opinion, came with the Internet. It also provided ultra-easy access to something that is fine as an occasional treat but hell for your health (in this case, sexual) on a daily basis.

Whether porn is good for us as a society isn't the point. I'm also not going to debate what does or doesn't qualify as porn. Even if there's no touching or personal contact (such as on popular sites like www.mygirlfund.com, where women post photos of themselves and can engage in video chats for a fee that they negotiate), it's still porn.

As long as sites like this become profitable, the porn genie can never be crammed back into the bottle (and sealed up, then thrown into the ocean where it should sink down, down, down to the bottom and stay).

When I say that porn is killing America's sexual behavior, I am not kidding, nor am I exaggerating. I see the detrimental and grave effects of porn on men and women and their relationships every day in my office, and I hear about it every time I go on the radio. I'm particularly blunt about this topic because I believe porn is the single, largest non-health issue that makes relationships crumble. It's harming every aspect of sexual health.

Believe me, after all the stories I've heard about porn over the years, I'm the last one to judge. I certainly don't believe that all porn is evil and that anyone who watches it is morally lacking. Porn in and of itself isn't necessarily bad. My stance is everything in moderation. The occasional use of erotica—whether online, video, or print—is probably harmless.

It may even help spice up your sex life if *both* you and your partner are interested in exploring that option occasionally, and you both agree on what you like and what makes you happy. If your partner can watch porn in moderation—and lots of men and women can because they don't need it to get aroused—then you can have a lot of fun with it. In fact, it's often so ridiculous that it's laughable. Anything that makes a couple laugh together in bed is all right with me!

Note, however, my use of the words "occasional" and "moderation." If you and your partner don't watch porn, or watch it once in a while and have a giggle and mutually satisfying sex while stimulating your own libidos, that's great. You don't really need to read this section.

But everyone who has to deal with porn more regularly needs to come to grips with the porn epidemic and, more importantly, porn addiction, which is far more common than most people think. I know that some women can get addicted to porn, but I haven't met any of them. By far, the overwhelming viewers of porn, and those who become addicted, are men.

Sex can become routine for a lot of couples, and men often

see porn as a way to add some spice to the routine. But when men turn to porn for variety and escape, they don't realize that they're actually putting their sexual and emotional health at risk.

As you read in Lesson 1, a man who masturbates frequently can soon develop erection problems when he's with his partner. Add porn to the mix, and he can become unable to have sex and then start allowing his fantasies to cloud his judgment. He can, unwittingly or not, start comparing you to the women he's viewing. Do you have the body of a porn star? (Who would want enormous breast implants?) Do you have the stamina? (Who would want to endure the endless pumping?) Are you willing to have multiple partners at the same time? (I sincerely doubt it!)

I recently read an article discussing the fact that if patients felt that their doctors didn't really care, their health suffered—even if they weren't really sick. During their appointments, they see their doctors bent over their laptops, clicking away and stashing health info in electronic medical records. The doctors don't even bother to lift their heads and lay their hands on the patient to assess what's really going on. Once that ability to engage the human touch is gone, you're in trouble as a doctor. It's the same with relationships. Pornography is the equivalent of electronic medical records. It isn't hands-on. It isn't real.

Or, to use a slightly less doctor-driven image, porn is the equivalent of a blow-up doll. She certainly isn't real. She's actually rather scary-looking. She can help a man get his rocks off, but who wants to have sex with inflatable latex when a real, live, wonderful woman is ready and willing?

What drives me crazy is that so many teenage boys have their first relationship not with a person, but with what they're watching on their computers. In all of recorded history, porn has never been easier to access. It's there with the click of a mouse, twenty-four hours a day, seven days a week, 365 days a year, and into perpetuity. With more than 420 million adult websites on the Internet, the wealth (if you want to call it that) of material is inexhaustible.

So how do you get through to the adolescent boy's horny, testosterone-filled brain that in porn, women are actresses—and usually badly paid ones at that? These actresses are pretending, and they will always say "Yes" and do whatever the man wants and have "orgasms" (the vast majority of which are fake), no matter what's done to them. Real teenage girls or women are never that acquiescent, nor should they be! Yet for boys who are just starting to date while trying to decipher the mysteries of the female (and *that* can take a lifetime), and who are shy and fumbling and anxious, porn can make them feel better about their fantasies and inexperience.

Porn allows them to think that if and when they're with a real woman, they can translate their masturbatory prowess into mind-blowing sex. But this is a short-sighted, erroneous way for these impressionable young men to behave. The only way to learn about women is to spend a lot of time with them. And the only way to get really good at having sex is by having real sex with real women. Porn can set these men up for very warped and hurtful encounters with women who won't ever play by the totally ludicrous rules of porn.

Watching porn is a passive experience—even if a man is masturbating to it, he is still watching other people on a screen going about whatever they're moaning about. And as such, porn creates its own universe. In this realm, sex takes place without any emotional connection because it is wholly a fantasy. It might look real and the actors might be having actual sex, but because they are actors, they are faking their feelings. They are spouting dialogue and doing what their directors and producers told them to do.

When patients discuss their porn viewing with me, I ask, "Which would you and your partner have if you had the choice? Sex with an emotional connection or sex without? Is it about porn, or is it about a real, live person caring about you?" My patients inevitably tell me that, of course, they want sex with emotional connection—but sometimes, in truth, they really don't. They just want to be alone with their porn and their masturbation.

So, yes, porn is a problem that's out of control. No data can get super-specific about the numbers and hours spent watching porn, because these statistics would be impossible to collect with any accuracy, especially because men tend to fudge, if not lie, about this topic. I tell my patients and their partners that porn viewing is an addiction when it affects your life or hurts a loved one, or both.

Look at the fallout from the actions of New York State politician Anthony Weiner. He is a sex addict and a narcissist with a compulsion to "sext," or send explicit photos of himself, to strangers. His problem is so bad that he had to give up his seat in Congress. After a public mea culpa and a decision to run for mayor of New York City in 2013—and just when polls showed he'd basically been forgiven—he was caught yet again, sexting to more women. His compulsion seems to be as intense as his denial that it's a problem.

Take this quiz and see if your partner might be at risk for porn addiction.

IS HE ADDICTED TO PORN?

☐ Do you know how much porn he really watches?

☐ Does he talk about porn a lot?

☐ Does he have particular favorites that he likes to watch repeatedly?

☐ Does he ask you to watch with him?

☐ Does he get angry if you don't want to watch with him?

☐ Does he withhold sex if you tell him you don't want to watch?

☐ Does he want to act out different scenarios he might have seen, even if you make it clear you don't want to?

☐ Is he asking for rougher sex or more unusual positions?

☐ Is he suffering from any ejaculation problems?

☐ Is he being more critical about your body, particularly your breast size?

☐ Is he asking you to make any changes to your body, such as getting a Brazilian waxing, that you are uncomfortable with?

☐ Does he *not* talk about porn a lot, even when you have your suspicions?

☐ Does he spend a lot more time on the computer that he won't talk about?

☐ Have you discovered that he has secret or password-protected sites online?

- ☐ Does he shut the pages down or instantly minimize them when you walk into the room?
- ☐ Or is he pretty shameless about watching it in front of you?
- ☐ Has he ever watched porn in an inappropriate public place (such as on an airplane)?
- ☐ Does he have another cell phone account?
- ☐ Are there unusual charges on your credit card?
- ☐ Will he cancel social engagements because he'd rather watch porn?
- ☐ Are his friends dropping hints to you about the porn he watches?
- ☐ Does he get up in the middle of the night to watch porn?
- ☐ Is he evasive or defensive when you ask him about porn?
- ☐ Does he choose porn instead of wanting to have sex with you?
- ☐ Is he having trouble at work because he's watching porn there?
- ☐ Does he get angry if he is unable to watch porn when he'd planned to?
- ☐ Have you found hidden stashes of porn magazines, DVDs, or flash drives?

If you answered yes to many of these questions, don't be in denial. Your partner has a problem with porn. A lot of women suspect their men are addicted to porn but aren't willing to accept the possibility and seek solutions. If this behavior has been going on for some time, you probably need to know the answers to these questions. Remember that a man is addicted if his behavior is negatively affecting your relationship. Find a neutral third party—an addiction counselor, not just a therapist—to help your partner or show him this book.

The ESP of Porn

Like many other things that are bad for us yet can taste good in the moment—like drugs and alcohol, junk food, and nicotine—pornography can start out as a harmless, once-in-a-while indulgence. But without even knowing it, a lot of men can get sucked into the vortex of a true addiction to porn that will be hazardous to their physical and emotional health.

Countless experts have discussed the shocking amount of porn consumed in this country, but I have yet to hear any of them talk about the overwhelming majority of men who watch a lot of porn and then find themselves with sexual *performance* problems.

These are sexual performance problems that can destroy your relationship.

Yes, something that is supposed to stimulate and arouse men (or women) sexually can actually destroy their overall libido and performance. So why isn't anyone talking about the effect on sexual performance—the ESP—aspect of porn? Probably because they flunked sex ed for grown-ups. They're discussing *why* a guy watches it—and not *what happens to his penis* when he watches.

I can tell how much porn a man watches as soon as he starts talking candidly about any sexual dysfunction he has. Guys who watch a lot almost always describe the porn they love in glowing terms, like it's their secret friend or (worse) their mistress. Some men go on and on, describing details about their favorite porn stars or different films and websites. Conversely, I rarely hear about their partner or spouse.

Some of my patients say that they're only trying to keep their penises healthy by frequently watching porn and masturbating to it. Yes, regular ejaculation is needed to keep the blood flow steady so a penis can function properly. And yes, regular ejaculation is also associated with a lower risk of prostate cancer. But the best kind of ejaculation is with a loving partner, not with a blurry computer screen that's streaming porn.

When a man chronically watches porn and gets off on it, or watches porn with his hands on himself so he can masturbate at the same time (which is what usually happens), the sensory stimulation he gets from the virtual world makes it much more difficult for him to get aroused, stay aroused, and be happily aroused by the real, live woman in his life. Namely, *you*.

In other words, his frequent, porn-fueled masturbation leads to sexual dysfunction with a partner. If he can only have an orgasm when watching porn, and if he becomes accustomed to having orgasms only in a certain way or while watching a certain thing, he's in trouble—and so are you. He should always be able to climax with his partner without needing any outside influences. Porn isn't just risky business; it's a killer for your sex life.

Dear Dr. Fisch: My Husband Is Taking Too Long in Bed and It's Getting to Me

Dear Dr. Fisch,

My husband and I have only been married for a year, but our sex life isn't what it used to be when we were engaged and when we first got married. I'm pretty sure it's him who's got the problem. Every time we have sex, I can have an orgasm pretty quickly, but it takes him about thirty minutes to have one, too. I know my husband sometimes watches a lot of porn, so is that the reason why he takes so long? I mean, we really love each other and I know he wants me to be happy with our sex life. He tells me the porn is harmless and he likes to watch it because it's "fun." What should I do?

Signed, Porn Is Harmless Fun, Right?

Dear Porn Is Harmless Fun, Right,

When men are porn addicts, they sometimes want more sex, not less—but they want sex on their terms to fulfill fantasies "inspired" by what they've been watching. The porn and his masturbating are having an obvious effect on your husband's performance when he's having sex with you—it's called retarded ejaculation. His lasting "too long" is the opposite of what most men experience when they watch a lot of porn—they can't last at all!

While lasting too long sounds like it could be a good thing, it can be just as troublesome for a relationship as when he's finished too quickly. I'm sure there have been times when you've gotten sore or bored or fed up, and wonder when he's going to get the job done. Not to mention that the constant friction can actually be painful after a while.

The first thing you need to do is tell your husband that you'd like him to cut back on the porn. If he balks, tell him it's only for a few days. Then don't have sex with him during that period. When a man doesn't ejaculate for several days, he will be a lot more sensitive (and a lot hornier!), and he'll be more likely to climax within a normal time.

Second, try to make your foreplay into more play. Ask him what he likes to do when he's watching porn, and replace his hands with yours. When you touch him where he likes to touch himself, he'll relearn how to get that same sensation when he's alone with you. Do this together—no cheating for him and going back to pornl—and I promise that he won't need thirty minutes for an orgasm any more.

What Porn Does to Your Head

Aside from leading to sexual dysfunction, porn can make men and women feel totally inadequate. The bodies on view are gleaming and perfectly toned. There's seemingly no mess, no muss, no wet spots on the sheets afterward. A man can pump and pump and pump, and the woman receives him with (alleged) ecstasy. She has no problem swallowing anything. She encourages him to act out in ways that you or your partner might find out of control or offensive. He has no problem sustaining an erection. They both have an orgasm in perfect synchronicity.

But the vast majority of this is fake or completely unviable. Porn sets you up to be disappointed no matter what. Adults who have had decent sexual experiences with loving sexual partners will be able to laugh off the moans and groans and pneumatically enhanced body parts because they realize how disconnected porn is from reality.

What's dangerous is that those with less sexual experience might not. When they watch, they're dissociating from reality. Because porn implants a certain idealized notion of what sex is "supposed to be," it can create unrealistic expectations. These can be very hurtful for anyone who doesn't manage to measure up (as if you'd want to!).

Dear Dr. Fisch: I Can't Have Sex Unless the Porn Is On

Dear Dr. Fisch,

I've been married to my wife, Sonia, for more than seventeen years and I love her very much. We have had a good marriage, but the problem is I know I'm addicted to porn. I'm really scared that Sonia is going to leave me. I can't say I blame her. For the last couple of years, I can't have sex with her unless the porn is on. She hates it but she puts up with it because she loves me. But she's finally reached the point where she can't stand it anymore, and she's about to pack her stuff and go. I need help. What should I do?

Signed, Need Porn Rehab

Dear Need Porn Rehab,

You already know you need to make a decision. Which do you want more in your life: your wife or pornography? You have to pick, right now, or you will lose her. Sonia is going to leave you if you keep doing what you're doing.

Watching porn as a couple can sometimes spice up a couple's sex life, but both of you need to be into it. Excessive porn-watching is like excessive drinking or gambling. It's an obsession and a compulsion, and incredibly harmful to your health and to your relationship.

What you have to do first is admit that you have a problem. Denial is a killer. Then you have to be honest about porn's effect on you and on your partner. Next, you need to do something else. Have sex with Sonia without porn, for starters. Then find something to occupy yourself during the time you usually spent watching porn. Just as smokers need to find something to do with their hands when they quit—drinking coffee, chewing gum, or eating (which is why ex-smokers often gain weight), you need to find a better substitute. Luckily, you already have one lying next to you every night.

If you pick porn instead of your wife—and I sincerely hope you don't—then your issues are beyond the scope of this book, and you and Sonia need to see a therapist to help you work things out. Look for one who specializes in addiction treatment. During

> your sessions, you will be encouraged to talk candidly
> about your behavior, fears, hurt, and anger. The thera-
> pist's role is as a neutral referee.
>
> Being able to talk honestly can improve communi-
> cation and intimacy. It'll take some time to repair the
> damage that's been done, but if you're both serious
> about making it work, you'll be able to get through
> this and have enjoyable, real sex again.

Is Watching Porn the Equivalent of Emotional Cheating?

I'm often asked if watching porn is emotional "cheating."

I wouldn't say it's *cheating*, because your partner is not having a physical relationship with another human being. But I would say that it's an emotional *impediment*. If, for example, your partner tells you he's going to go read while you're doing something in another area of the house and you walk into the room twenty minutes later to find him watching porn, you have an issue that needs to be discussed. And if your sex life undergoes any changes due to his porn habit, action needs to be taken.

So I understand why I'm asked this question. It's easy to worry that your partner doesn't love you any more if you suspect he's fantasizing about someone else during sex. Or that he's sizing you up and finding you wanting, no matter how much he denies that.

Still, a lot of men would rather masturbate to pornography than go through the work of maintaining a deep and loving emotional connection to their real, live partner. The irony is that men really want to have intimate relationships. That's what human beings do. We're social creatures, and we need love and companionship. Of the thousands of men I've seen in my practice, I can think of only a handful who are "confirmed bachelors" and really don't want to settle down and live with a woman.

But as you know, it's easy to fall in love or lust. It's a lot harder and takes a lifetime of determination—to follow the guidelines you'll read about in Part II—to maintain a wonderful, loving, stable, thriving, and endlessly evolving relationship. Men who don't want to do the work, or who need to address their deep-seated fears and insecurities about relationships, and the men who choose to use porn erode or evade these connections.

Dear Dr. Fisch: I Found Porn on My Husband's Computer

Dear Dr. Fisch,

Can you help me? I am freaking out. Yesterday, I found a lot of porn on my husband's computer. Justin told me I was overreacting, but he's full of it. We haven't had sex in a while, like maybe twice a month, and he admitted he masturbates when he watches the porn. Of course I'm wondering if his cache of porn might have something to do with why we're not having sex. Justin denies it, but I don't know what to believe.

Signed, Rated R, Not NC-17

Dear Rated R, Not NC-17,

How do you know when your partner is looking at too much porn? When it starts affecting your relationship. I'd say that's the case here. Having a great sex life is all about communication. A man who's busy watching porn rather than being with you is never going to be able to communicate with you, and you'll never have great sex with one another, if you don't take action. You guys are only having sex twice a month, and Justin is admitting that he masturbates to the porn. That's not great sex. That's masturbating sex for him and no sex for you!

Try establishing a schedule around when you'd like to have sex. Pick two days a week that are set aside just for intimacy, not for porn. This means Justin can't watch porn on those days. Make sure you really plug into what each of you wants in bed.

I'm sure you have certain fantasies you'd like Justin to project onto you, so go ahead and explore these fantasies without indulging in porn. If you want Justin to make you dinner, he should do this. If you want fore-play, I'm sure he'll accommodate this, too. Or if he wants you to dress a certain way, be open to his suggestions.

Dealing with Porn Addiction

Porn addiction is like any other addiction. It can easily ruin the addict's life and the lives of those around him. It can cause your partner to morph from a reliable, responsible, emotionally con-nected man to someone you don't recognize anymore. It can cause intense shame and despair, because admitting to a sexual compul-sion is extremely difficult, more so than with drug or alcohol addic-tion, because it's considered far less acceptable. Porn addiction can be so all-encompassing that it can cause your partner to lose his job; if he is publicly exposed, even worse for him and his family.

How does anyone get over a porn addiction? It's not easy but it is doable. Have your partner try these steps first:

- Take a break from the physical habit of watching porn. Turn off all devices with porn stashed on them, and destroy or throw away any hard copies of porn on DVDs.
- Try to schedule something absorbing during the time you usually spend watching it. If you can take a short trip, great. (Just don't turn on the TV in your hotel room, where porn is available.) Even better if you have children along because you won't want to be watching porn with them nearby. Or do additional chores around the house (like the long-overdue garage cleaning, painting, or gardening—something that is physical and impossible to do around electronic devices).
- Try not to masturbate for a few days. Then you should be much more ready to have satisfying sex with your female partner.
- Talk about how much you love each other, and how much you cherish the emotional aspects of your sexual relationship so you can refocus on the qualities of your partner that you first were attracted to. Act the way you did when you were first courting—I'll bet porn was not part of the equation then. This way, your desire will build naturally so that you both can enjoy the pleasure of real sex and leave the virtual sex to the robots.

If this doesn't work because your partner is truly addicted or unwilling to discuss the matter with you, or both, you should consult professional help. Look for a sex therapist experienced with porn addiction and sexual dysfunction. Be prepared for the addict to have a hard time. If addictions were easy to kick, there wouldn't be any addicts.

Dear Dr. Fisch: Porn Is My Girlfriend

Dear Dr. Fisch,

I'm thirty-six and addicted to porn. I watch it every chance I can get—at home and on my cell phone even when I'm out in public and someone can see it accidentally. I've dated a lot so I'm not really lonely, but I've never had a serious relationship, which I'd like to do. What can I do to cut porn out of my life to achieve that?

Signed, Dial P for Porn

Dear Dial P for Porn,

First of all, I'm glad you've admitted that you have a problem with porn. That's the first step to solving it. The reason you've never had a serious relationship with a woman is because you're already in a relationship with porn. It sounds like porn has taken over most aspects of your life, so there's little room for much else. You say you're not lonely, but I'm doubtful that's the full truth. Most men your age have already been in a relationship deeper than just casual dating or hook-ups.

You've already taken the first step toward dealing with your addiction by being honest about it. Next, it's time to get help. Addictions like this are hard to beat on your own, but with professional help, you can over-come them. So I strongly advise you to see a health-care professional with expertise in sex addiction.

If it makes you feel better, you are not alone in this. Did you know that porn addiction is the *number one issue* that sex therapists deal with? This realization will also help if you want to develop a social network—there are support groups for people struggling with sex addictions that can really help. And, at least for a while, you may have to get rid of any porn videos, programs, websites, and apps on your computer, cell phone, or tablets so you don't get tempted to open them again.

You can do this. Get the help you need to beat this addiction, restore your self-confidence, and get your life back, and then you'll be able to have a strong and com-mitted relationship with a woman who'll love you back.

The Bottom Line about Porn

Watching porn and masturbating is the sexual equivalent of fast food. It's instant gratification, and it's fine once in a while when you're craving some french fries or nachos smothered in that fake, orange cheese goop, but for nourishment? Forget about it.

Having great sex with a partner you love is the equivalent of a five-course meal cooked by a master chef. Creating and serving the meal is going to take a lot more work. But it's going to entice all your senses. It's going to smell and taste delicious. It's going to make you feel terrific (unless you're like me and feel guilty for eating a huge slab of cheesecake for dessert!). Eating it is going to be a lot more fun and a lot more memorable.

Once a man understands the potential consequences of eating a lot of fast food laden with salt and fat and sugar, he knows that it will make him sick. I hope that men addicted to porn will also realize that watching actors and actresses pretending to have pleasurable sex can make him, his partner, and his relationship sick, too.

His Cheating Heart

Take this quiz, and if the answers stack up, you already know what's going on. I haven't met a woman yet who was wrong when her gut told her something shady was going on with her partner.

IS HE HAVING AN AFFAIR?

☐ Does he suddenly want a lot more or a lot less sex (when there are no compelling reasons for this, such as illness or stress)?

☐ Is he working unusually late or taking more business trips than usual?

☐ Is he incommunicado for long periods?

☐ Does he spend an inordinate amount of time on the computer or other devices?

☐ Has he suddenly become more interested in working out and losing weight (when he might have balked before)?

- ☐ Is he wearing a new cologne or suddenly paying attention to scent or a grooming routine?
- ☐ Is he shaving more often than he usually does?
- ☐ Has he expressed interest in changing his wardrobe all of a sudden, with no clear reason?
- ☐ Does he mention wanting to take up a new hobby, again with no clear reason for it?
- ☐ Is he overly affectionate or far more affectionate than normal (and it feels fake)?
- ☐ Is he finding fault with everything you do, all of a sudden?
- ☐ Do you feel like snooping through his papers and email because you don't trust him?
- ☐ Does he look secretive when the phone rings, or is his cell phone behavior unusual?
- ☐ If you ask him point blank whether he's cheating, does he get really angry and defensive?

How Can You Tell If He's Cheating?

If you answered yes to many (or hopefully not all) of the questions in this quiz, it's time to get tough with yourself because the issues and your fears about them are highly unlikely to go away on their own.

I had this conversation with an acquaintance when he confessed his cheating ways to me not long ago.

"Who answers the phone at your house?" he asked me.

"Anyone but me," I said with a laugh. "I hate to answer the phone, and I know someone's going to pick it up."

"Well," he said smugly. "The guys having the affairs are the first ones to pick up the phone. They might be afraid someone's calling that they don't want their wives to know about."

Of course, now that everyone is hardwired to their cell phones, a man who's cheating can simply buy a prepaid cell phone to cover his tracks, right? Digital technology has made it easier than ever to cheat. Worried about a mistress calling the house? Get a prepaid phone that is virtually untraceable. Worried about how to meet someone who is discreet? Go to websites like www.ashley-madison.com, whose motto is "Life is short. Have an affair." Or go on regular dating websites and lie about your marital status. It happens all the time.

And it isn't just men cheating on women. Recent studies have shown that 45 to 55 percent of married women and 50 to 60 percent of married men have extramarital sex at some point during their relationship. And that's just for married couples. Couples who aren't married are even more likely to have an affair.

As Jerry Lee Lewis said, there's a "whole lotta shakin' goin' on."

So why do people cheat? "The bottom line regarding infidelity is that men are cheating on their wives primarily for sexual reasons, while women are cheating on their husbands for emotional reasons," said Ruth Houston, infidelity expert and author of *Is He Cheating on You? 829 Telltale Signs.*

My take on it is that men cheat because it's easy, it's quick, and it gives them a thrill. It reaffirms some men's masculinity, and others have narcissistic tendencies that make them feel they can do whatever they want without consequences, simply because it makes them feel physically good (if only in the moment of instant gratification). In other words, men often cheat because they can when the opportunities arise. Women cheat because something is lacking in their relationship—closeness and intimacy, time together, LSD (listening, security, and desire)—or because something has been done to them. For example, they've been cheated on or have experienced withdrawal by a partner.

Cheating always raises a complicated welter of emotions. These are extremely painful emotions triggered by betrayal, lying, dishonesty, duplicity, unexpected feelings for another, and sexual difficulties.

Luckily, many of the issues that can cause so much frustration in relationships and that can lead to cheating are preventable (especially once you and your partner master the LSD you'll read about in Part II). It's so prevalent and you may know many couples who've done it, but that doesn't mean cheating has to become part of your world, too.

Some couples can use cheating as the wake-up call they need to finally assess and deal with the good, bad, and ugly in their relationship. Maybe the cheating was done out of boredom or anger or curiosity. Maybe it was just a stupid, selfish mistake in the moment that caused intense guilt and shame and will never be repeated. Couples who can get everything out in the open and deal with duplicity with honesty and courage can sometimes manage to push past the pain, forgive, and move on to a stronger and more loving relationship.

Is Cybersex Cheating?

Just as I'm often asked if porn viewing is emotional cheating, so am I asked if cybersex is cheating.

Cybersex is cranking online porn up a notch, because during

a cybersex session, the participants are having virtual encounters with each other, via a computer or other device, to send and receive sexually explicit messages or images. This usually includes masturbation by one or more participants who get turned on by these conversations and images.

While cybersex is physically safer than real sex—no touching, no diseases, no getting caught if you're in a restaurant or club or hotel—it still involves a lot of thinking, talking, and acting out with another person. So whether cybersex is actually "cheating" depends on your personal definition of "cheating." Is it physical cheating? No. Is it an emotional *impediment*, a word I referred to earlier in this lesson, or is it emotional cheating?

My take on this is that anyone who is having live encounters with another person, whether online or in the flesh, is involved in some degree of "cheating."

I don't necessarily consider it "cheating" if you fantasize about other people while you're masturbating. Many people do that, both men and women. However, lots of the men I talk to use that notion as a diving board to launch themselves into the cybersex pool. They rationalize their cyber sessions as being merely a bit more *juicy* because they're masturbating in real time to a real person—but still someone who is a "stranger" and with whom they don't have an emotional attachment. Or so they claim.

And that's when the problems start. What started out as a diversion can quickly shift into a more complicated relationship, especially if the cybersex sessions become more frequent and more graphic and more demanding. (I'm not even going into the possibility of getting caught sexting on a work phone or computer, which can wreak havoc on professional reputations.) Having fantasies about the cyber object of affection can interfere with regular sex with a partner as well, if not make it impossible. That's when the *impediment* has become full-blown emotional *cheating*.

Dear Dr. Fisch: What Really Counts as Cheating?

Dear Dr. Fisch,

I'm thirty and so is my husband, Walter. We've been married for seven years and have four young children. I want to know what counts as cheating. I think cheating should include things like texting and social media like Facebook, as well as sexual infidelity. Walter doesn't agree. He tells me that since he's more experienced sexually—because he used to "cheat" on his other girlfriends before we got married—he knows what cheating is.

He says that having sex with another woman is the only thing that counts as cheating. But I know he's still sending emails and texts and Facebook friending and messaging other women all the time, even though he thinks I don't know this. He can spend hours doing it on weekends when he should be with me and the children. I am very worried that this is going to ruin our marriage and that Walter is ready to walk out the door to be with one of these women he says he's not involved with. So who's right?

Signed, Want to Go Offline

Dear Want to Go Offline,

First, something is very wrong with a husband who is messaging other women behind his wife's back. People think cheating is just having sex, but emotional cheating is very real, and I'm afraid Walter has a bad case of it. He needs to understand that his communicating with other women is still a form of a relationship. He can deny it all he wants, but what he's doing is cheating. And you're right, because this can be a marriage-wrecker if it continues much longer.

Walter needs to man up and take responsibility for being a good husband as well as a good dad. A man who is cheating emotionally can destroy his family just like a man who's cheating physically can. Believe me, the kids know when there's tension in the house and Mommy and Daddy aren't getting along.

Kids grow up fast. Walter isn't going to want to look back ten years from now and realize that he missed their childhoods and doesn't know his own kids because he was too busy having virtual relationships with women other than his wife. Or that they're angry and resentful at him for all the problems his selfishness caused the family. He needs to think about what kind of role model he wants to be for them.

Walter also needs to disengage from what is clearly a social-media addiction. If he's spending an inordinate amount of time online, as you said he was, then he's addicted. It's his drug of choice right now. And if any kind of addiction causes a problem in a relationship—and this one clearly does—it's time to give it up.

He also needs to listen to and acknowledge your hurt feelings, and how he's making you feel vulnerable and insecure. Show him the facts in this book!

You have the right to know that your husband is going to be there for you emotionally, physically, and financially. In this particular situation, he needs to tell you that, yes, you are correct that he is "cheating." Whether he likes it or not, he's emotionally involved with these other women, and if this marriage is going to be saved, he needs to cut it out and cut them off.

I think you both would benefit from couples' counseling. Having four children in seven years can stress out any couple, no matter how loving the marriage. But managing the stress and the worries isn't a license for a man to run away from his responsibilities by cyber-chatting with other women.

STIs: How to Protect Yourself

Here's how to never get a sexually transmitted infection (STI): Never have sex.

Or, during your entire life, only have sex with one partner, who is a virgin the first time you have sex.

Or, insist on going with any partner to have a full blood workup to check for all communicable diseases prior to having sex, so you can verify the results.

Now that those fairly unlikely ideas are out of the way, here's a more helpful hint: Always use protection unless you are certain that your partner is disease-free.

STIs are on the rise. The American Sexual Health Association has some sobering statistics on its website (www.ashastd.org/std-sti/std-statistics.html). They claim that "more than half of all people will have an STD/STI at some point in their lifetime." And that "recent estimates from the Centers for Disease Control and Prevention (CDC) show that there are 19.7 million new STIs every year in the United States." That is an awful lot of bad news and devastated people.

What's even more worrying is that STIs are often asymptomatic, which is one of the reasons they can spread so easily. Some are irritating but don't put your health at risk. Herpes, for example is relatively benign and highly treatable with medication, unless you are pregnant, as it can be transmitted to the baby during childbirth. Other STIs, like chlamydia, can cause pelvic inflammatory diseases and infertility in women if they are not treated. Still others like HPV (human papilloma virus) can cause cervical cancer. HIV and hepatitis can be lethal themselves or lead to fatal complications if left untreated.

When you are sexually active, it's important to be honest with your partner. This can be hard to do, especially if you've ever had an STD or STI. (See "How to Bring Up a Delicate Topic" on page 195 for tips.) If he doesn't want to discuss this topic, or if you feel he's not telling you something, you may want to reexamine how much you can trust this man. Particularly, can you trust him enough to shed your clothes and have sex? If you feel you're at risk (maybe your partner had an affair), ask your doctor for a screening at your next checkup or ask him to get tested. Always use a condom unless you have the utmost trust in your partner.

Dear Dr. Fisch: My Girlfriend Doesn't Like That I Work in a Strip Club

Dear Dr. Fisch,

I'm a DJ in a strip club and it's a great job. I make a lot of money and I can play the music I like, and I have a lot of fun. When I started working there, I was interested in dating the strippers. But once I got to know them, I realized they weren't for me as girlfriends or lovers or whatever, because most of them are addicts or work as prostitutes after the club closes, or both. I mean, I am not trying to insult what they do, but I don't want to go out with anyone who does that kind of stuff.

Besides, I have a live-in girlfriend named Julianna, and we're in love and everything. However, she doesn't like that I work in the club and that some of the strippers are platonic friends. She says that even if they're addicts or hookers or whatever, I'm still around naked women every time I go to work, and she doesn't trust me. She doesn't believe that I'm being faithful to her. How can I make her understand that I'm not cheating on her and don't want to leave this job?

Signed, Please Don't Stop the Music

Dear Please Don't Stop the Music,

I hate to say it, but this relationship doesn't sound like it's going to go very far. It's great that you love your job and are a friend to your colleagues at work, and that you're trustworthy and dedicated to Julianna.

You're certainly not cheating—far from it. But working around sexually active, naked women all the time is going to be threatening to your girlfriend—and most other women. Women want security. Maybe they want children and a home. You have to accept the fact that your unusual job is going to make any relationship you have more difficult.

For now, all you can do is be straight with your girlfriend. Tell her why you like your job and why it's important to you. Maybe she could come to work before hours and meet some of the strippers and see how they talk about you in a brotherly fashion.

Acknowledge her feelings—put yourself in her shoes—because you probably wouldn't love it if she worked all day in the company of handsome and naked men! If you can resist temptation and she can raise her trust level a bit, the two of you may work things out. But you may end up having to choose your job or your girlfriend.

Just Can't Get Enough: Sex Addiction

People are not just addicted to porn. They can become addicted to sex, particularly when for them it's all about the sex act and orgasms to the detriment of everything else in the relationship. Given how easy it is to become infected with a sexually transmitted disease such as HIV, sex addiction is not just a problem. It can be lethal.

Sexual addiction, or "sexual dependency," is a valid psychological disorder. It's hard to treat because no single behavior pattern defines it. A sex addict can suffer from compulsive masturbation, compulsive and chronic porn viewing, compulsive heterosexual and homosexual relationships or affairs, compulsive cybersex, prostitution, exhibitionism, and voyeurism—and even progress to such heinous crimes as child molesting, incest, or rape.

Like any addiction, sexual dependency is a compulsive behavior that dominates the addict's life. The addict will continue to engage in the addictive behavior despite clear harm or distress to himself or those around him. Sexual addicts make sex a higher priority than everything else in their lives. (If you think that sounds a lot like porn addiction, you're absolutely right!) They are so driven by the addiction that they can sacrifice their family, friends, work, and health to keep having sex. They seek the orgasm as a compulsion, as an immediate gratification without the emotional connection.

On my radio show, I often get calls from men who are spending all their money on prostitutes or strip clubs. I ask them if they can pay all their bills. If they can't pay the mortgage because they've spent all their money on erotic massages, they have an out-of-control addiction. If they admit they've been going to prostitutes for ten years, they know what they're doing wrong without me telling them.

But if a man can afford to fund his addiction, is he still addicted? Of course he is. He's a *functional* addict. Does he need treatment? That depends on how adversely the addiction is affecting his life and the lives of those around him. A rich single guy who chooses to spend his money on prostitutes is making a choice about how to spend his money. It's not the same kind of problem that a rich married guy has if he's doing the same thing.

In other words, anything that adversely affects your partner's life or your life is a problem. I have a very low tolerance for alcohol, so if I drank one glass of wine every day I'd be an addict. But I know plenty of people who can have two or three drinks a day without getting drunk or having it affect their ability to function at work or with their families. Are they alcoholics? Not by my definition.

Sex addicts need to admit that prostitutes and porn stars can't ever really care about them, even if they do a great job of pretending. But a man in a committed relationship who hires prostitutes or goes to strip clubs either doesn't care or is deluding himself. He wants the quick rush of pleasure and of having a (paid) woman do everything he wants to his body. If he's a narcissist, he also will feel that he deserves this side activity for whatever reasons he tells himself. (His wife doesn't like anal sex. She doesn't give him as many blow jobs as he wants. She expects to have an orgasm during sex. She wants intimacy—and so on.) If these habits become ingrained, after a while they become the norm. That's when the addiction usually starts to spiral out of control.

When you're having sex, the goal is not just to have an orgasm. The crucial point of sex, beyond the physical gratification, is to build powerful emotional connections and love. Those are the keys to the best and most satisfying sex a person will ever have. Sex addicts need to understand that the real pleasure is in support, comfort, love, and security in their committed relationship—not in the sexual gluttony of mindless one-night stands.

This kind of powerful sexual intimacy can be incredibly tough to sustain over the years, which is one of the reasons why people cheat. A few sex addicts can overcome their addiction on their own (just as some cigarette smokers can finally kick their habits), but far more need professional counseling. Anyone who has problems controlling his or her sexual urges needs to seek competent professional help as soon as possible.

The addict shouldn't be ashamed to admit he or she has an addiction, although this seems harder for sex addicts than for alcohol or drug addicts. That's because the shame level is so high for sex addicts, who may also have to deal with the ignorant or judgmental stance some of their loved ones or colleagues take.

A woman who finds out her partner is sex addicted should never blame herself, even though I've lost count of how many women have told me *they* feel guilty about the problem. They wonder if they've done something wrong and "driven" him to it. I have to reassure them that this is rarely the case.

The most important question a sex addict needs to answer is: Do you want to have a relationship with a real person? This relationship needs to be more important than a transient orgasm with a stranger. Because the only way to get away from sex addiction is to be able to have a relationship in which you care for somebody and want to make him or her happy—and that somebody cares for you and wants to make you happy, too.

I hope that knowing more about the tough stuff that can go wrong with relationships actually makes you feel better. What I mean is, if you are experiencing any of these issues, you are not alone. Turnoffs, bumps in the relationship road, disagreements, bad habits—all the stuff that happens to every couple—are all part of life. How you deal with them is what counts. Read on, and let a little LSD make you and your partner a whole lot happier.

PART II

COMMUNICATION 101

Learning How to Say What You Need

"Turn on, tune in, drop out" was the famous phrase of American psychologist Timothy Leary. Back in the Swinging Sixties, he was doing research at Harvard on the effects of psychotropic drugs like LSD. Yes, that Harvard, and yes, that LSD. Eventually, Leary got fired because his love of LSD went a little too far, but I still love that phrase. Except I've reshaped to it to fit my relationship-improving system:

- Turn on your partner, and he'll turn you on even more... once he knows the essence of good listening.
- Tune in to each other's needs, especially the one for security.
- Drop out of boring, unsatisfying patterns and drop in to desire.

In other words, the essence of my favorite form of LSD is: Listening + Security + Desire. This is the kind of emotional "drug" that will keep your sexual and emotional relationships happy and thriving.

Trust me on this: You can forgive someone for any number of faults when the sex is really good, but after a while, the reality of every other aspect of your relationship is going to set in. The morning after eventually arrives when the glow of the sex the night before has faded, and with it comes the need for LSD. Desire is delicious, but you still need the listening and the security or the desire can ebb away really fast, leaving frustration and regret.

Having a great relationship means you have one thing above all else: the ability to show your partner that you care about him. In this part of the book, I'm going to show you how to teach *him* to show you how much he cares about your life together. This is what **LSD** is all about: Women want men **L**istening to them + they want to feel **S**ecure + they want to feel **D**esirable. The man in your life needs to:

- Get better at **Listening** to you. By doing so, he will validate what you need to talk about. He has to stop interrupting. In Lesson 5, you will see how that means "shut the fuck up."

- Provide **Security**. By doing so, he will make you both feel safe and able to conquer the world. In terms of financial security, he needs to get a decent job and not be a bum, making the effort so that you and your family will hopefully have financial security now and in the future. Even more important, however, is that he gives you emotional security so you feel safe in his love and physical security so you feel safe in his arms and together in your home. What could be better than returning from work every day to a home that is your haven from the ups and downs and zigs and zags of life?

- Fuel your days with **Desire**. Women want to feel desired, so he needs to be lavish with compliments, acknowledging the effort you put into your appearance and everything you do. Women really want men to make them feel they are worth it. Because, naturally, you are!

Doesn't that sound almost ridiculously simple? Or rather, impossible? Actually, using the LSD system in your relationship is deceptively simple. Most of the couples I see have been married for years, and I see how they behave with each other. They love each other, but they can't express what they need in bed and from each other. They have absolutely no language to do so. That's because they honestly don't know anything about sex—what's normal and how to explain their desires.

At the heart of all of the relationships I see in my office or hear about on the radio are two people who each just want to be acknowledged for—and accepted—the way they are. But they are rarely willing to put in the work to compromise and accept the other as is, although the women, who are usually more attuned to their emotions and capable of talking about them, are almost always more willing than their partners are.

If a man is frustrated because his wife won't have sex with him, he may boast, "I'm just gonna go out and find somebody else." I believe him. Does he care? Sure—about himself. About his marriage? Not with that attitude. Will they stay married? Only if they both start communicating!

That's exactly what I'll show you to do in the following lessons. Once he finally starts listening, the more he'll give you the security you crave, and the more he'll understand your desires—which will jump-start your ability to communicate, in bed and out.

LESSON 5

L IS FOR LISTENING
...SO SHUT THE F**K UP

You can't have security and you certainly can't have sustained desire if you can't communicate with each other—and communicate *well*.

That may sound obvious, but you wouldn't believe how many couples don't stop to think about whether they are communicating, what they are communicating, and most importantly, *how* they are. If you don't know how to listen—and, equally if not more importantly, if your man doesn't know how to listen—you'll never get anywhere in bed (or out). You'll always be talking *at* each other, not to each other. You'll be frustrated. You'll think more about what's *not* being said than what *is* being said. When this happens regularly, it can doom even the happiest of relationships. This lesson will help you get back to basics—to the L in LSD: Listening.

Four Little Words Every Man Needs to Tell Himself: Shut the Fuck Up
Communication = Listening

I'm a lucky guy. I'm happily married to the world's greatest woman, but if somebody would have told me thirty years ago what I know now about how to communicate in a loving relationship, it would have made a lot of difference over the decades we've spent together. We would have fought less. My wife, Karen, would not have been so frustrated when I'd try not to roll my eyes and say, "I can't take it anymore," practically every time she wanted to talk about something for any length of time (in my male view, "endlessly").

Most of all, I would have understood my wife when she was talking to me. Before I figured it out—or rather, before Karen helped me figure it out!—she'd talk about things I thought I didn't want to hear. She would talk about work, what happened with the kids, what happened when she was shopping, something that needed work around the house, her girlfriends' relationships, you name it.

But really…I just didn't know how to listen.

Yes, I was a typical guy. Mr. Macho Me thought I was too important to take time to really *hear* what she had to say. The truth is I didn't know *why* I should listen. After all, wasn't what I said or thought more important than what anyone else had to say? Even if it was said by my beloved wife?

Fast-forward to now, and my twenty-year-old daughter helps me to remember why that arrogant attitude had to disappear. She'll say, "Let's take a walk, Dad," and we'll go out and she'll talk. Okay, so sometimes (all right, a lot of the time) she goes and goes like the Energizer Bunny, but you know what? Over the years I've grown accustomed to listening to her, and she knows it. (I'm not just a better listener to *her*, but to *everyone*.)

Even better, I really like hearing what she says. She's smart and funny and interesting. She has all the passions and convictions that young women should have when they're finding their place in the world, and it's exciting to share that with her. In fact, the best conversations we'll have are during this special time together. Everything she needs to say comes out—because she trusts me to listen.

If my daughter had gotten the message from me, as many daughters do from their dads, that I was too busy and self-important—canceling on school events or family outings I'd promised to go to because "something came up," or talking too much about my work and not asking enough about hers—to take the time to let her talk, we would not have become as close as we are.

She'd have a much harder time confiding in me, and I wouldn't know what's going on in her world. She'd shut down to me. She would blow me off for time with her friends if I wanted to spend an afternoon with her. She wouldn't accept my opinions as having much validity. I know that we could have started fighting, leading to tension in the house—with her and with my wife. All because I would have been too selfish to listen.

This point came across loud and clear the other day when a friend was complaining about his wife. "All she wants to do is talk," he grumbled. "What's the matter with her?"

"*Nothing's* the matter with her," I replied. "That's the point."

"Are you insane?" he asked. "You know what she's like. She just goes on and on and on, and it drives me nuts."

"Nope. I'm not kidding. And let me tell you what to do the next time she's talking."

"What should I do?"

"*Shut the fuck up.*"

His jaw dropped open. "Are you freaking kidding me?" he asked.

I shook my head and laughed. "No, I'm not. The real problem here isn't your wife's chattering. *You* don't know how to listen. One of the simplest, yet most difficult things a man can do to foster togetherness is to simply listen to his wife. And stop making faces—really, this isn't as trivial as you think it is."

Of course this was when he started rolling his eyes.

"Once you figure it out and you do start listening," I continued, "you're gonna be amazed at how much better your relationship will be. Better communication, better understanding, and much, much better sex."

Of course, that is when he stopped rolling his eyes.

It's a simple but crucial point. The more a man can listen, and listen well, the more his partner will know that he's there for her, that he isn't surreptitiously texting under the table, for example, or thinking about the game on TV when she's looking for understanding and sympathy. His loved one will be happy to be acknowledged and feel cared about, and that often translates into vastly improved communication and happiness when you're having sex.

You're not going to want to have sex when you feel your partner couldn't be bothered about you. But you will want a lot of sex when you're perfectly attuned to each other, listening to and acknowledging what each of you has to say. As I've found out over the years with my wife—as well as with all the couples who've come to me as patients—a deepening of intimacy, security, and desire becomes rooted when a woman knows the man in her life is truly listening.

But there's an even bigger point: Once you start listening and the woman you love knows you're listening for real, *she won't talk as much*. She won't need to! Your conversations will become more economical, more succinct, more comprehensible, and a lot more loving. You won't be at cross-purposes, arguing over every little thing. She won't be bottling up frustration at you or your relationship and then feeling the need to let it all out in one long spew that leaves you both hurt, confused, and angry.

When you feel like your partner truly listens to you and pays attention, you also find it easier to let go of a lot of the little things that bothered you before. You won't need them as ammo any longer. You'll joke more and fight less. You'll get what each other is saying.

This doesn't mean, of course, that you won't mess up sometimes and really let each other have it. All couples fight, even the happiest and most devoted. Fighting once in a while can be productive if it clears the air and allows you to get your feelings out or resolve an issue that has come up. Nobody can go through life in a state of mellow bliss, avoiding all arguments and never once raising his or her voice.

While constructive fighting ends with resolution, leaving you both feeling more connected and having more faith in your relationship and your ability to work things out, destructive fighting doesn't allow you to appreciate your overall happiness or to grow together and continue to strengthen your bond. But once he's better at listening, your fighting spats and episodes will go way down. Why? Because you will have prevented the same old arguments about the same old topics from even coming up. He will have acknowledged who you are and what you need and what you are saying. He will make you feel loved. And that is a potent aphrodisiac.

A man who knows how to listen is going to have a much happier, healthier, and more satisfying sexual relationship. That is why, when I'm talking to male patients or callers on the radio, I often joke, "How do you know when a woman is finished talking? Her lips stop moving."

Call me crass—it doesn't matter. Men get the joke (and yes, it's a *joke*!). They laugh. Sometimes they laugh a little too hard. They know what I mean. Because they know, deep down, that they *don't* know how to listen.

They're so used to not listening to their wives or girlfriends that they think this is how things work. That not listening is acceptable for men. They just don't get it.

That's because they haven't reached the point in their relationships where the word "communication" isn't just about he said, she said. Good communication between partners is a bedrock for a healthy relationship—especially a sexual relationship, because if you can't say what you want, how will you ever get it?—and for overcoming a wide range of challenges in all aspects of your life together, whether they're about sex and desire, raising the kids, or who takes out the garbage. Good communication is also one of the most difficult things to do well in a relationship, especially for men.

For women, it's simple. You listen and then you respond, and then you listen some more and then you respond again. Women are by nature more in touch with their emotions and have had years of practice doing this with their girlfriends, family, and colleagues. This facility with emotional intelligence helps women foster openness in all their communication and an instinctive ability to know when to speak and when to listen.

Your ears are finely attuned to pick up subtle communication skills, to assess body language, and to hear what others are saying and process it, even if you don't like what's being said. Because you've been listening well since you were a child, this skill is now as simple as breathing. It's just part of your nature as a woman.

But just as women can't understand why men have such a hard time listening, men can't understand why women have so much trouble keeping their lips zipped. That's because men aren't innately able to maintain or stay invested in the natural give-and-take of conversations that comes more easily to women. They just aren't.

Are there stats to prove that men don't listen? A study done at the University of Sheffield in the United Kingdom and published in the journal *NeuroImage* discovered that men have to work harder at listening to women because their brains process the sound waves of speech differently. Men use the part of the brain designed to hear music, not voices. (This means he can blame his listening problems on basic physiology, so I suggest you don't mention this study to him!)

I'll push past this anatomical quirk and say that men basically don't have a clue. You may also have learned from personal experience that they are far less skilled than women at opening up and coping with the emotional aspects of relationships, especially if the guy is dealing with a male sexual problem. They are less emotionally intelligent than women and approach problems from a more analytical, "how-can-I-fix it?" point of view. But that doesn't mean that men can't learn more effective ways to promote harmony in a relationship.

So it's up to you to teach the man in your life how to listen. You need to teach him that listening is a skill, like learning how to surf or ski, close a deal, cook a steak to perfect doneness, or change a diaper.

And what's the easiest way for a guy to learn how to listen?

By following this simple rule: *Guys—shut the fuck up.*

For guys, this doesn't just mean to shut your mouth and let her talk without being interrupted. It means shut off the running commentary in your head while she's talking—the silent commentary that she can tell is going on when you look at her with blank eyes and ask, "What did you just say?"

You'd be surprised at the number of subtle ways in which the listening problem can manifest itself. Here's an example of a typical couple in my office—typical because he doesn't listen and she is totally frustrated.

Chloe and James were sitting opposite me. Chloe was making full eye contact with me, while James was busy inspecting the window blinds. Before I'd even opened my mouth, James's body language had signaled to both of us—but mostly Chloe—that he'd tuned out. His posture was rigid, and he had shifted sideways in his chair to look out the window, practically turning his back on his wife. Then he slumped even further. This was tantamount to saying, "I'm not interested, and I don't want to hear it." Talk about shutting down the conversation before it even started!

Swift action was required. Simply by assessing their body language, I could tell that this couple had no idea how to have a conversation. Their pattern started with each person stating their opinion. James didn't listen when Chloe was talking, and she knew it. She felt dismissed and he got annoyed. They both were vexed and frustrated, and that started a fight. It was almost as though a visible wall hovered between them.

I looked down at their paperwork. Chloe was on the fertility drug Clomid and had been through a series of inseminations. She was worried that the clock was ticking and needed advice—and some hopefulness.

Chloe sighed. "I really want to have a baby," she said, looking right at me.

"Here we go again," said James.

"Should we continue the inseminations, or move on to in vitro?" she asked.

When a woman wants to have a baby, she's super motivated. Now more than ever, her husband or partner needs to listen to what she has to say. Did James understand this? Obviously not.

"She wants to have the baby too quickly," he said, still looking out the window before meeting my gaze. "I don't know why we're rushing. We've only been married three years."

Notice how Chloe and James were not talking to each other—they were talking to *me*.

"We're *not* rushing," Chloe said as her eyes filled with tears.

"Why don't we wait?" James retorted. He glanced down at his cell phone.

"Look," I explained, because I know all too well that infertility can be an extreme test for a relationship, and a man who doesn't understand this is lost and risks losing his partner, too. "I always say 'wait' is a four-letter word when it comes to having children. I never say wait to a woman who wants to have a child, because a woman who wants to have a child wants to have a child *yesterday*. If you don't know that yet, it's time to start listening to your wife because she's driving the car—and she's driving at one hundred miles an hour right now. You are going to have to learn to listen to her or suffer the consequences."

"Don't I have any say in this marriage?" James said.

"No," I replied. "When it comes to having a baby, not at this time. What I mean is it's her body. So yes, in theory this is a joint decision, but when a woman really wants that baby, it's going to become an overwhelming focus for her. Her clock is ticking, and that's a valid tick because her eggs won't last as long as your sperm can."

Chloe and James looked at each other.

"Does James interrupt you a lot?" I asked Chloe.

"Absolutely," she replied.

"So what?" said James.

"When do you guys talk?" I asked.

"We never talk," Chloe said. "I try to bring up how worried I am about not getting pregnant and he doesn't care. He says he's too busy, but I know he's not listening."

"That's because she talks too much," he said unkindly.

"Well," I went on, "when that happens, I immediately tell the man in the room to sit up and turn to his wife. That's a great start. The next step is to let her have her say and to *not* interrupt. Look her straight in the eye, and look at her lips if you're having trouble following, but just listen without interrupting. She doesn't want to hear your opinions right now. She just wants to talk it out."

Chloe nodded vigorously while James rolled his eyes. She didn't see him, but I did.

Take a look at their dialogue again. Chloe was stating what she wanted (a baby). James had tuned out. He was busy thinking about what *he* wanted, not understanding that part of the deal when they got married was to have children. He was dismissive to her, bordering on rude. I had a feeling that they never properly discussed when to have children before they got married. Chloe might have thought her desire was crystal clear, but with James so bad at listening, it didn't matter now how much she'd stated what she wanted then.

This scenario and similar ones have happened many times in my office. The man sits in the chair, looking out the window and not even acknowledging that he's not listening. Sometimes he interrupts and sometimes he silently sits, bored or seething or frustrated, or all three. I've never had a wife say, "You know, honey, thanks for not listening to me." Why would she? He knows he's not listening. He's just never been told *how important it is that he shuts the fuck up!*

So how do you get him to talk? I wish there was a one-size-fits-all answer. Sometimes you just can't. That's the case with men who go past not listening. They tune everyone out so much that they become experts with the silent treatment. That's a communication emergency, and you need to call Relationship 911. (You need professional counseling to get to the root of his inability to talk to you.) It's hard to believe a man cares about his partner if he's so unwilling to talk to her. That's so fundamental that no relationship can survive without it.

For most people, it's much easier than that. Here's how I resolved things with Chloe and James. First, I taught him the basics on how to listen that you'll learn in the next section.

And then I added, "When you leave this office, I want the two of you to go to a restaurant, and I want you to sit in front of each other without any distractions. You need to look at each other when you're talking. You need to talk about having a baby. And you, James, need to keep it zipped when Chloe is telling you what she wants."

I wish I could say that James looked sheepish at their next appointment. He didn't, of course. He's a typical guy, and he's not going to admit that he was wrong. But he did say, "Okay, I get it now. It's such an obvious thing. I understand what I need to do." He sighed. "And we're going to keep trying for that baby."

Learning How to Listen

The idea of men not listening is such a well-worn cliché that a commercial on TV for Klondike ice cream bars used this notion to get a laugh. In it, a couple is sitting on a sofa. She's talking, and he's looking at her while mentally doing a five-second countdown. After five seconds, he wins an award for listening to his wife. For all of five whopping seconds! And what is this commercial called? "Five Seconds to Glory: Good Listener."

Clearly, Klondike thought this was a concept that would resonate with their demographic. I'm telling you about it because it does ring true for a lot of women. So before you start teaching the man in your life how to listen, remind yourself that this is not going to be about immediate gratification. Teaching him how to do this will take time.

Remember, this is most likely a new skill for him. Not only that, but for most men (unless they grew up in a house with a dozen sisters), it's one that doesn't come naturally. It's not as instinctively easy for him as it is for you. Listening without interrupting can be incredibly difficult for men because, as I said earlier in this section, their brains literally don't process sounds the way women do, especially in the heat of an argument or emotionally loaded discussion.

The goal of his learning how to listen is to allow you to say what you want to say, no matter how sensitive or emotional the subject, and no matter how off-base, illogical, uninteresting, or even wrong it may seem to him—at first.

That doesn't mean, of course, that you can go on and on about whatever you want and expect a captive, silent audience at all times. (Listening and good communication goes both ways.) It just means that you can use that to establish the boundaries for the healthy back-and-forth that is the essence of good communication in a loving relationship. You have a chance to speak, and then it's *his* turn.

Guy Rules for Listening

Here are a few rules for men on how to be great at listening:

- Pay attention to what she is saying. Do not just nod and say umm-hmm. She'll know if you've tuned out.
- Look at her when she is talking to you. *Do not*, upon painful risk of being denied sex for the foreseeable future, ever look down or away at an electronic device when she is talking to you (unless the caller ID identifies the call as a true emergency, and no faking allowed). Also, do not look down at her chest or any other part of her body—or out a window or around the room, no matter how nice the view might be.
- Do not interrupt.
- Repeat: *Do not interrupt.* Yes, you. Shut the fuck up!
- If you feel you are about to burst from not talking, count

silently in your head to ten (or twenty, fifty, or whatever number it takes for you to stay quiet) until the impulse passes.

- Or try deep breathing. Breathe in for a count of five, and then breathe out for a count of five. Keep doing this until the impulse passes. (Try not to breathe too audibly, so you don't sound like you are sighing impatiently.)

- Or try sucking in your abs when you do this and concentrate on holding the movement for a few seconds. Not only will it help you not talk, but it will improve your core strength!

- Men who are reading this section because your wife or girl-friend just shoved it under your nose, trust me that it helps to try to at least *pretend* that you're listening. After all, you expect them to listen to you. After a while, you may surprise yourself. You actually *will* be listening, and you might even start hearing things that are interesting. And trust me, that will lead to better sex and more of it.

- Understand that women don't necessarily want or need their partner to jump in to solve their problems or suggest ways to fix things (as you'll learn in the last section of this lesson). Most of the time, they just want their partner to listen to what they have to say and try to understand with-out passing judgment. Resist the temptation to interrupt or debate. That doesn't mean not talking at all; it just means giving a woman the time to finish her thoughts completely before you respond.

- If you're still having a hard time listening, remind yourself that you already know how to listen, because you probably do it all the time with others. At work, for example, do you interrupt your boss or supervisors when they're telling you about a big project? Of course you don't, because you know the rules and don't want to get fired. Do you interrupt your colleagues when they're describing an important task at a meeting? Of course not, because you know the rules and want to succeed in your career. Pretend your partner is a client, colleague, or boss (in many ways she is), and treat her with the same respect. Remember that what works with your career and your colleagues will work wonders at home with your partner, too.

For both of you: Realize that it's equally important to check the instinct to get mad if your partner's response isn't immediately what you expect (usually for women) and the instinct to try to solve the problem quickly (almost always for men). (See the last section of this lesson, starting on page 198.)

Listening Is Like Practicing Poker

What makes a great poker player? Not just the ability to count cards and make risky bets—but his or her ability to "read" the other players to get clues about what's in their hands. (These often subtle yet deadly giveaway clues are called "tells.") A poker player with a terrific sense of who's bluffing is a poker player who's going to win.

Body language is an incredibly important component of great listening. When couples come to see me, I immediately get a sense of what their relationship is like by how close they're sitting to each other, whether they are shifting around in their seats and moving away from each other, and whether there is mutual eye contact. I have to figure out whether what I'm being told is the truth, or whether one or both of the parties is bluffing.

So if your partner likes to play poker or any other kind of game that involves bluffing, have him practice on you. Make it a game he'll want to play. Have a conversation and ask him to rate what you're saying as truthful or bluffing. Believe me, he'll be looking very closely at your face, and he'll be listening intently. Then use this opportunity to say to him what needs to be said. Don't let on that you're using these training sessions to get him to finally listen with undivided attention to what you have to say!

Strategies for Breaking Old Habits and Creating Healthy New Ones

Here are some suggestions for men to ingest, memorize, and use so they can improve their listening skills, and make their partner feel loved and understood. You can also use them as a refresher course for yourself, because they apply to both of you.

More Guy Rules for Better Listening

- Stick to "I" statements—statements that express how you feel or think about something your partner has said.
- Stay away from "you" statements. Don't accuse, and do *not* distract her or derail the conversation by throwing in something unrelated that bothers you about your partner.

- Use reflective listening techniques to clarify what is being said. You can say, "I hear you saying…" and paraphrase what your partner just said. Ask if what you said is correct. This can help you avoid misunderstandings and demonstrates that you really have heard what your partner is saying. It also allows you a minute to gather your thoughts to respond respectfully.

- Avoid talking about sensitive or difficult subjects when either of you is extremely tired or stressed, or both, which always exacerbates any conversation difficulties. This is one of the most basic rules, yet many people use the most stressful time of the day to bring up something that will push buttons. (It reminds me of toddlers having tantrums. Many of their meltdowns happen simply because the child is tired and hungry.)

- Never have an important conversation when either of you is under the influence of alcohol or some other substance that makes it harder to control emotions.

- Don't make threats or ultimatums if your partner has mentally checked out or picked up his or her iPad. Let it go for now, but make it clear that the conversation will continue when you are both not so stressed and tired.

- If you feel "stuck" in a disagreement, back off, cool down, and remind each other of the core values you both cherish about each other and how much you love each other. If this doesn't work repeatedly and you can't get unstuck no matter how hard you both try, it may be worth seeking out a neutral referee such as a therapist or counselor who can help you both.

- When a woman is talking, *she doesn't want to be fixed.* A lot of men are in the problem-fixing business. They want to treat their relationship partner the way they'd treat a business partner. But what works professionally should stay in the office. In a *relationship*, men should not decide to fix the problem unless their help is solicited.

In other words, don't try to fix something that doesn't think it's broken. If she wants a fix, she'll ask you for a fix. The worst thing you can do while you're listening is to tell her what you're going to do, or what you think is the way to fix the situation. She doesn't care what you think at that particular moment. Maybe she'll care later. That's not the point. The point is: Shut the fuck up, leave her to fix it on her own, and listen.

In addition, if your wife is talking to you about tulip bulbs the cat dug up in the garden, that's just as important as what *you* want to talk about. Understand that a problem she thinks is worth discussing is worth it, whether it's small or monumental. So if you say, "Why are you talking to me about this?" I promise you there will be no sex that night.

Most of all, realize that in relationships, if the woman isn't happy, nothing's going to happen in bed. Nobody is going to have sex if they're not happy with the person with whom they're having it.

Think of this as the Italian cheesecake rule. I am fairly good about watching what I eat, but my downfall is the Italian cheesecake at my favorite neighborhood restaurant. Every time I go in there, I swear I'm not going to get a big, fat calorie-bomb slab, and every time I end up scarfing one down. Why? Because it's fun.

Because I love it. Because eating it tastes great. So great, in fact, that it's worth the extra workouts or my wife rolling her eyes at my lack of willpower.

So when people ask me, "Why am I not having sex?" the answer is easy. If you enjoy sex, you'll have it more. If you're not having sex, somebody does not like something about it, and that something could easily be your behavior. If women don't like their partner's behavior or they don't feel loved and *heard* by their partners, they don't want to have sex. Want to have more sex? Make your partner feel loved and attended to. This isn't rocket science, guys.

Getting back to the cheesecake, remember this: great sex is like a meal. There's the appetizer, the main course, and dessert.

Your relationship itself is the appetizer.

All this talking and the communication is foreplay. It may sounds as unsexy as listening to your accountant tell you about your taxes. Really. But when done right, good communication is the all-important emotional foreplay before the physical foreplay of lovemaking.

Next comes the main course: the sex itself. And then dessert is when you're smiling and satiated.

Dear Dr. Fisch: My Boyfriend's a Stink Bomb

Dear Dr. Fisch,
  My boyfriend refuses to shower and he really stinks. I've told him practically a hundred times and he ignores me. I can't believe he thinks it's okay, but he claims that

he can't smell anything and no one else has told him there's any stench. I don't want to sleep in the same bed with him, much less even think about sex. It's disgusting. What can I do to get through to him?

   Signed, Soap Lover

Dear Soap Lover,

   Women want to be listened to, they want to feel secure, and they want to be desired. That's the essence of my version of LSD. When your boyfriend refuses to shower, he's not listening to you. And when your boyfriend doesn't listen to you, you don't feel secure or desired by him. Plus, who wants to touch someone who smells rank? I wouldn't.

   Here's what might help: tell him you are getting naked and into the shower, and you would really love it if he got in there with you. I will be very surprised if he turns down such a luscious invitation. Be sure to have some deodorant soap in hand when he gets in, and give him a good scrubbing. This will be the cleanest foreplay you both will ever have!

   If he still balks, that may mean that things aren't supposed to work out between the two of you. Your self-respect is at stake here, so see if he'll listen to you before making any more decisions. If he isn't willing to clean up, try to find a man who has better hygiene and a greater willingness to listen to common sense and common courtesy!

*Let Men Practice Their Listening Skills without **You***

Guess what—your partner's practice time on listening skills is not going to be with you.

If you've tried and tried and *tried* and just can't seem to get conversations to work, it may be time to back off, cool down, remind each other of the core values you both cherish, and then, if needed, take the discussion to someone who can mediate as a neutral party and with whom your partner can talk and listen. This can be a therapist or counselor, a trusted member of the clergy, or even a friend or family member who knows you well and whose advice you can trust to be neutral and positive.

Even if he is driving you so crazy that you've vowed never to have sex with him again, try as hard as you can to give your partner some space to talk things through with someone else. Especially if it has to do with sex. Like my wife, you may have been talking to your girlfriends about dating and sex and boy talk ever since puberty, but boys just don't talk that way. (That's the reason I'm writing this book—men don't know who to talk to about sexual issues and communication issues and women issues!)

I think it's incredibly sad—and ironic—that most men avoid talking with other men about the topics they really need to communicate on. They find their concerns, especially if they have to do with erectile problems or infertility or their libido, too embarrassing or shameful to bring up. They don't know how to get started. They walk into my office with such fear and trepidation that I really feel for them. After I make them feel safe enough to open up, they walk out feeling relieved and reassured that their fears were acknowledged and their concerns understood.

They also often have learned the value of having a conversation about a difficult topic without being interrupted or dismissed.

But if these guys don't have a doctor like me to talk to, who will they talk to?

I always encourage men to talk to a brother, a father, a best friend, a physician, or a clergy member about what they're going through. It is comforting to be heard and helpful to air your feelings away from your partner. Tell your partner I said so. Once he starts opening up about his own challenges, he'll discover that getting it all out can be refreshing and liberating.

What Women Never Want to Hear from a Man

They never want to hear the blunt truth about how they look, unless they specifically ask him to be blunt. And even then, be very careful.

If a man says, "That dress looks a little tight on you," or "Have you gained a few extra pounds?" bullets will come after him.

It may seem obvious, but many guys don't get this. Gently but firmly let him know that he cannot ever tell a woman she looks fat. Women are not looking for honesty; they're looking for reassurance that they're still attractive and appealing.

What He Should Say Instead

Teach the man in your life how to give compliments that may skirt the truth yet are not flat-out lies. (The latter can be patronizing or demeaning, especially if a woman knows they're said just for the sake of giving a compliment.)

A woman will nearly always be flabbergasted (and thrilled, of course) if a man tells her, "You smell delicious." Or, "I love that dress. It really suits you."

This is an incredibly simple technique that reaps enormous rewards. Why? Because a sincere compliment shows that a man noticed something unique about a woman, that he thought about it, and that he took the time to tell her that he noticed. It also makes a woman happy that he appreciates her appearance, making her feel more confident and sexy. That glow can last all the way into the bedroom.

Women Need to Listen, Too—and Cut to the Chase

As hard as it can be for women to admit sometimes, they aren't always perfect communicators—even when they might think they are (but don't worry—nobody is!). Often, the larger issue for women is that they think they've expressed their needs well when they haven't. In other words, they shouldn't expect their partners to be able to read their minds.

Strategies for Breaking This Habit and Creating a Healthy New One

If you want or need something from your partner who you feel never listens to you, try some of these strategies:

- Find a time to talk when he isn't deeply preoccupied with something. For example, don't try to bring up something you feel is important to discuss during the Super Bowl or after he's had a terrible day at work (unless it's an emergency that truly can't wait).
- Speak up and speak simply. State your point right away. Don't use a lot of sentences when one or two will suffice.

- Don't give a long preamble or make excuses. Just cut to the chase.
- Even better, stick to just a sentence or two. Every man can pay attention for one sentence. After that, he may start checking out. And if he checks out and you know that he's checked out, you will find that infuriating. A conversation that could have been short and sweet and productive turns into an avoidable "You never listen to me" argument. And I know you don't want that to happen!
- If you think he still hasn't gotten the point that you made in one sentence, repeat it. With the same short sentence. This is key, especially for men. Whenever I give a lecture, I repeat my main point three times—at the beginning, in the middle, and at the end. I tell everyone what I'm going to talk about; I bring it up again in the middle; and I recap it at the end. The repetition helps to make the point stick. Expressing your needs to your partner is the same thing. State your needs, be concrete, and don't be shy about repeating if you need to (as long as it doesn't turn into a long, drawn-out nag that defeats the purpose of the conversation).

Jackie and Andrew were a perfect example of this. They sat in my office glaring at each other. Or rather, she was glaring at him and he was busy looking out the window. (Does this sound familiar?)

Jackie: He doesn't want to commit. We've been together eight months. I want to get married, but there are certain issues…
Me: Well, tell me about your sex life. Is it great? Is it good?

Jackie shrugged and looked at the floor, embarrassed. Andrew yawned. I knew what that meant. It meant that neither of them knew how to talk about sex.

Me: Did you ever talk to Andrew about it?
Jackie: No, I didn't speak to him about it, but you know I want him to be more aggressive during sex.

As soon as she said that, Andrew's eyes lit up and he eagerly turned to her.

Andrew: You do?

Jackie nodded, and the floodgates opened. They were then able to talk about their needs and desires and fantasies. I knew that they'd be having a lot of fun together later that night—and in the years to come. Jackie realized she couldn't blame Andrew for not making her happy when she wasn't able to tell him *what* would make her happy!

Remember, keep it simple and keep it positive. Don't tell him, "You don't know what you're doing. I told you to do it this way last week. You're not listening to me," because that will deflate a man quicker than a punctured beach ball. He will tune out and get defensive.

Instead, say, "I love it when you _____." Such as, "I love it when you take charge," or "I love it when you let me get on top."

How to Bring Up a Delicate Topic

Delicate topics are never easy to bring up. This is something I deal with daily in my practice, and it's an important aspect of how I treat my patients. When I was younger, doctors kept secrets from their patients, and patients often kept secrets from their loved ones. Cancer often wasn't mentioned even when people were dying, for example, which deprived those sufferers of the chance to deal with their mortality and put their house in order. And as you know, secrets are lethal in any relationship.

When I have bad news for a patient, I never come out and say, "You have Stage IV prostate cancer, and your chances for survival are slim." Instead, I say, "I have the pathology results, and six of the twelve markers show cancer, but cancer can be treated. There are plenty of options, and we're going to explore all of them. I'm here for you, so let's talk about it." That's much easier to handle, and it still tackles the real issue. Otherwise, the person's anxiety becomes unbearable and that can be harmful to them, too.

Whenever you bring up a delicate topic, don't just present the problem. Be ready with solutions—even if you're not sure they're going to work. A solution can be as simple as handing him this book and saying, "Here, take a look at what Dr. Fisch is saying about this issue. I'm so relieved that it's nothing too serious and we can work on it together."

When delicate topics are unavoidable, these tips should help:

- Try to avoid this discussion when either of you is very tired or very stressed. It will always go better if you've both had a decent day, and you're not hungry or frustrated or exhausted. An ideal time is when you're out to dinner and able to talk to each other without interruptions.
- Think of setting up the conversation as the foreplay of the delicate topic.

- Men are concrete thinkers. That means you need to prepare for a delicate conversation with the facts. Do your research ahead of time. For example, if his problem is premature ejaculation, do some reading (like in this book!) so you know how common it is, which will help you with the conversation. Then you can say, "Dr. Fisch said that _____, and I agree with him."

- If you need help remembering what to say, write it all down and refer to your notes. Don't tackle more than one or two issues at a time. Then say, "Honey, I've been thinking about this, and I wrote down what I think would make our lives fantastic."

- Don't go into a long explanation first. Come right out and say it quickly. Cut to the chase, such as, "By the way, I was thinking…things could be fantastic in bed, and here's a way to make our sex lives more fantastic." Then tell him what it is. That is a much better strategy than saying, "Our sex life stinks."

- Always be positive.

- Frame the conversation with compliments. If, for example, he's been perfunctory at best in bed lately, say, "Sex is the barometer of a relationship, and I think the sex we have could be better." Or, "I read in Dr. Fisch's book that a different sex position might be a lot of fun. I would like to have sex this way, so let's try it."

- Don't put off the conversation. Nobody wants to hurt someone else's feelings, especially those of your partner. But if something is wrong and you don't spell it out, it can't be fixed!

Sometimes, men just need an opening. Like Robert. He had an affair, regretted it, and went to counseling to see if he could repair his marriage. I asked him, "Did you tell the therapist how often you have sex with your wife?"

"I haven't had it in a year," he said.

"So did you tell this to the therapist?"

"No."

"What are you waiting for?" I encouraged him. "Bring it up!"

That opened the floodgates. Robert confessed to straying because, in large part, he'd been so sexually frustrated but didn't know how to talk about it. His wife didn't realize how important sex was for him as they'd gradually stopped having it over the years and she thought he just didn't want it anymore. Neither of them ever brought it up. If they hadn't finally talked about it, they might have gotten divorced over a lack of communication, not because they really wanted to.

Is This You? Catching Bad Communication Patterns

Now that you have some strategies for teaching your partner how to listen, take a look at these "he said, she said" conversations and see if you recognize yourself in any of these patterns. Be honest. I know that I can talk like this. A lot. *Everyone* talks like this from time to time. We can't help it—it's just human nature. But if you find that one of these is your pattern—or if you partner agrees that this is his pattern—at least you both know it. You're aware.

That's great. Acknowledging what you aren't doing well is the first step toward figuring out how to fix things.

Ashley and Bill: When Juvenile Just Doesn't Cut It

Bill and Ashley have been together for a year and are both happy sexually, but they always seem to disagree—and the fighting can sometimes be juvenile. For instance, sometimes Bill pulls Ashley's ponytail while she's driving or calls her a booger or fart face. Ashley is getting fed up with his juvenile attitude, especially because he blows her off when she tells him to cut it out.

Bill: You're the cutest little booger ever.

Ashley: I really don't appreciate you calling me that.

Bill: Why not? I said you were cute.

Ashley: I like that bit, but not the booger.

Bill: But you are a booger.

Ashley: I said, cut it out!

Bill: Oh come on, I was just teasing.

Their pattern: Ashley asks Bill not to do something, and he doesn't listen. He does it anyway. He thinks his need to be cute is more important than her asking him to stop it. He doesn't understand why it bothers her so much when he likes it and thinks it's funny.

My advice: Bill's insecurities are lending a juvenile tinge to his behavior, and I have to wonder why he feels compelled to do this. Often it's because the person is insecure about something or uncomfortable talking about some issue. Of course, some women like being treated this way, but Ashley had made it abundantly clear that she is not one of them. The dynamic that exists now may be impossible to change, in which case they may both be better off in another relationship. But it's equally possible that this could be one of those crisis points that can lead to new insight, changed behavior, and a better relationship.

I think Bill is having trouble listening and talking openly about how he feels. He hides behind the cutesy crap because he doesn't feel comfortable having normal communication about adult subjects. Bill's juvenile way of communicating shows contempt for his partner's sincerity, maturity, and feelings. This is a bad sign for the future of the relationship. Bill needs to try acting more romantic and grown-up. He can start by telling Ashley how much he loves and cherishes her, and he can say it with conviction. Then perhaps she'll stop seeing him as an immature little brother, and more as her protector and source of security.

If Bill can learn to take Ashley's feelings seriously, listen to her honestly, and talk openly and maturely about his own feelings, there is hope for them. But they both have to be willing to communicate. Stop with the name-calling and hair-pulling. If Bill likes to use terms of endearment, they should decide on one together that Ashley likes hearing. Anything will be better than booger or fart face!

Alexandra and Roberto: Talking at Cross-Purposes

Alexandra and Roberto have been married for twelve years and have three children. They are a perfect example of a couple in which each person has strong feelings about what they want, but they don't know how find a middle ground. As a result, Roberto has stopped listening to Alexandra because he's convinced she won't ever give in, and they're both angry and frustrated. I asked them how often they wanted to have sex.

Alexandra: Maybe three times a week.

Roberto (laughing): Oh sure. I want that, too. And more.

Alexandra: We're not having any sex because I don't want to have another baby.

Roberto: Here we go again.

Alexandra: You're not listening to me.

Roberto: No, you're not listening to *me*.

Alexandra: No, you aren't. I've told you a million times that I am not going on birth control because the hormones screw me up, so you need to use a condom.

Roberto: And I've told you a million times that I am not wearing a condom. That's for people who aren't married. I hate how they feel. If you cared about me, you wouldn't ask me to use them.

Alexandra: If you cared about *me*, you'd understand why I can't go on birth control.

Their pattern: Alexandra and Roberto are stuck and need a better way to communicate so they can solve the problem. They tune each other out because they both know they aren't going to reach any resolution.

My advice: This couple clearly loves each other, but they have no idea how to bring up a delicate topic. Instead of focusing on the problem, they need to focus on the solution. They both need to compromise, but arguing and not listening has been easier than sitting down and calmly strategizing about what to do. Alexandra can do her research by seeing her gynecologist and exploring birth-control options that don't involve taking hormones. Roberto can help her do this. Then he won't need condoms, which will improve his sensitivity, and she won't have to worry about getting pregnant or side effects from hormones.

Kelly and Ron: Three's a Crowd

Ron is still friends with his ex-girlfriend, Julia. Kelly doesn't mind them being friends but thinks Julia has crossed the line a few too many times. Julia works for Ron and somehow thinks this gives her license to show up at Ron and Kelly's house all the time. She still has keys and has gone so far as to throw out food Kelly has cooked. Kelly is upset and angry, but Ron thinks the whole situation is funny and that she's acting crazy. This makes her even more upset. Kelly wants Julia out of the picture, but Ron claims he needs her to help with his business.

> **Kelly**: But why is she still here?
>
> **Ron**: What are you, jealous?
>
> **Kelly**: No, I'm not jealous. There's just no reason for her to have keys to our house.
>
> **Ron**: You *are* jealous. I can tell.
>
> **Kelly**: Come off it! She's your ex and I'm your damn wife! I don't want her in my house!
>
> **Ron**: It's my house, too.

Their pattern: Kelly states her needs over and over again, and Ron ignores her or taunts her. Beyond not listening, he's actively dismissing his wife by ignoring her pleas.

My advice: This isn't about Ron wanting to have sex with Julia. He doesn't. What he seems to be missing is the valid point that Julia continually crosses the line, intruding on their relationship and actively undermining Kelly. Kelly has reasonably stated over and over that she doesn't like it and wants it to stop.

For this marriage to be saved, Ron needs to cut ties with Julia. Frankly, he is being an idiot by listening to his ego, rather than his wife. How would he like it if the tables were turned and she had an ex-boyfriend—with a set of house keys, no less—working in his home all the time?

The only mature way for Ron and Kelly to handle this is for Ron to give Julia notice and make her find another job. She will have to hand over the keys, and he should change the locks. Julia should also be forbidden from coming into the house. She will be able to find another job. Her employment is not something that Ron is responsible for, and frankly, his business should not be more important than his wife under any circumstances.

When I told Kelly to tell Ron how she really feels, this is what she said:

> **Kelly**: I can't take this anymore. You need to get rid of Julia or I'm leaving.
>
> **Ron**: Okay…I hear you. If you really want her gone, I'll let her go.

Hopefully, Ron will follow through. But the fact that he was so willing to allow Julia to continually cross boundaries that should never have been crossed makes this couple an excellent candidate for marital counseling. Allowing an ex to interfere with your current relationship is not a recipe for a successful marriage, and Ron's dismissive attitude toward Kelly makes it unlikely that they will last as a couple.

The "I Need Five Things during Sex" List

Like any good skill, learning to listen takes time, but it's equally important to become comfortable saying what you want or need so the other person has something to listen *to*. While you and your partner are exploring the strategies in this section, try this simple exercise in expressing what you'd like to have done to you in the bedroom. It's much easier if you take time to think about things and then write them down, however you want. Because you're in complete control, this also will help you push past any self-imposed barriers if you're having trouble expressing yourself.

1. Get out a pen and a piece of paper. Not a computer, cell phone, or any other digital device. You need to write, not type, this properly. This helps slow down your thinking and allows you to concentrate.
2. Divide the piece of paper in half. On the left, write five things you love about your partner.
3. On the right, write five things you want or what you'd like to do or have done to you during sex.
4. Show this list to your partner *before* you plan to have sex. (Nothing will kill the mood quicker than you whipping out this list when he's about to pop!) Ask him to read it aloud. Watch his eyes light up, especially when you tell him you are planning to have lots of fun doing all the things on the list with him. Then get busy!

LESSON 6

S IS FOR SECURITY
...SO THINK ABOUT WHY YOU'RE TOGETHER

What do couples argue about? Not just sex.

Money.

Money...and who takes out the garbage or changes the diapers or empties the dishwasher or mows the lawn.

Yep. Money and chores make the marriage go round. Whatever your financial situation, money is almost always going to be a huge component of your relationship.

Basically, we need to feel safe and secure. We need the emotional security of knowing that the person we love loves and cherishes us back, and that we can count on him or her no matter what.

And we need to be able to talk about money.

This isn't crass. It isn't about dollars in the bank. When I talk about money, I don't mean that couples need to be rich. Far from it. Financial security comes in many forms. A woman can be the primary breadwinner, and if her partner provides the childcare or something else that works for their relationship, I say fantastic.

For me, true security comes when a man knows he can make a woman feel secure enough that worrying about money is not going to interfere with their emotional security. Some of the happiest couples I know have limited means. Having gazillions in the bank isn't important to them. They cover their overhead and save a little when they can, but they're in it together, full partners in all financial decisions. That loving and trusting partnership extends to all aspects of their relationship. Believe me, I know a lot of very wealthy people who would give anything to have that kind of ease and comfort with each other!

The big problem is that couples are often no more able to talk about money and finances than they are about their sexual needs. Honestly. People don't know how to talk about money any more than they know how to talk about premature ejaculation.

If you're unable to talk candidly about both—because financial security is a need that must be brought out into the open—it can kill even the most enduring romance. And talking about money can be as difficult as talking about porn addiction or having an affair.

This is why the S in the LSD is for Security.

You can't have great sex without it.

If You Don't Feel Safe, Kiss a Fabulous Sex Life Good-Bye

Proof of this came from Carlo. He came into my office wearing tight jeans, a tight shirt, and a huge pair of blinged-out Gucci sunglasses. I jokingly put them on, and they practically covered my whole face. They were so heavy that I could barely keep my head up.

"Why do you wear these?" I asked.

"I wear them on the beach because I can't wear any other bling, and women think I have money," he said matter-of-factly.

I had to laugh at his flagrant faking.

But at least he was admitting his ruse, one as old as… Well, I'm sure the ancient Egyptians needed to feel secure, too. Those burial chambers weren't just to placate the gods. They were to prove to the living where the bling was.

I've lost count of the number of couples I've seen who are married, sometimes for a short while and sometimes for decades, and faking it. I'm not talking about designer sunglasses—but fake relationships. These are couples who don't have sex or who have bad sex. They may have loved each other once upon a time—or loved what they thought the other person was going to give them—but they sure don't seem to like each other.

Why do these couples stay together? Because the pain or aggravation of being together is less terrifying than the fear of being alone. Their need for security is overpowering their need to be happy and have great sex.

Never was this point more poignantly demonstrated than with a patient who's sixty. He started dating a fifty-five-year-old woman, divorced as he was. As soon as he came in, it was evident there were tremendous problems associated with this relationship

"Can you give me a prescription for Viagra?" he asked, looking sheepish.

"Why do you think you need it?" I asked.

"Well, my girlfriend is kind of bossy."

"How long have you been going out?"

"Three months. And she's been the controlling type from day one," he admitted, looking even more sheepish. "So, sometimes I'm having trouble…you know."

Yes, I knew very well.

We started discussing his options, and as he went into more detail about this relationship, he confided that they'd started going to a therapist.

My jaw dropped.

"You've only been dating for three months and you're seeing a therapist already?" I blurted out.

"I know, I know," he said. "But do you know how hard it is to meet somebody I feel a connection with? She has the same kind of background as me, so at least we have that in common. I just don't want to be lonely."

I really felt for this guy. He'd rather be miserable with a shrewish woman—so incompatible with his nature that he couldn't get it up—than be alone. I tried to convince him that if he stayed with someone who already made him so unhappy, he'd never find someone else who was a lot nicer—and with whom he'd have a more confident, thriving sexual relationship. Happily, he was able to break it off and keep dating. I reminded him many times that there were an incredible number of lovely women in New York City and he just had to take the time to meet them.

Men aren't the only ones who can be their own worst enemies. I also felt for a woman I know professionally. She's in her mid-thirties, super-smart, lovely, incredibly accomplished financially, and looking for a man with whom to share her life. She wants a husband. She wants children. And she can't find anyone to date. Why not?

"Because I can only go out with men who are richer and more accomplished and more successful than me," she said.

In other words, she is only willing to give up control to a man who makes her feel secure. She believes that she wouldn't be able to relax enough with a man who's her financial inferior—certainly not enough to let her guard down so she can have great sex.

I understand what she really meant. Women know that part of having sex is giving up control. If you're going to do that, you want a man who is secure enough in himself to know what he's doing, right? After all, what's sexier than a man secure in himself?

Many men who are just starting out in their careers or switching careers or starting up a business may be low on liquidity. But if they have confidence in their ability to move forward in business, as they do in all aspects of life, that confidence is a huge turn-on. Unfortunately, this woman's need for financial security beyond her own is likely to keep her single and unhappy.

I know plenty of men who are sexually and emotionally confident and who would be great partners for her. They just aren't rich enough for someone as well-off as she is. So while I admire her candor—at least she won't waste time dating men she knows won't make her happy—her specific need for security is devastating in its limitations.

Hopefully, if she hasn't yet met someone who fits her too-narrow criteria, she will let go of that fantasy and have a child on her own, or realize that her demands may be unrealistic and let her guard down long enough to meet someone incredibly loving, rich or not. That's what's really important, after all.

Creating Security: How Do You Show That You Care?

What do all secure couples have in common? Not big bank accounts. They have *trust*.

Without trust, there can never be security. Without security *and* trust, you can't have the best sex of your life.

In a good relationship, you trust that your partner loves you, is truthful, is faithful, and is there for you when you need him. The truest measure of character is not how people act when times are good and everything is easy, but how they do when times are bad, when they are stressed to the max and exhausted and worried. I've found that people enduring dire situations (death of loved ones, loss of their homes, loss of jobs leading to desperate financial straits) will pull through as long as they have the support of trusted loved ones who make them feel emotionally secure.

We all have basic security needs, and each person also has idiosyncratic needs depending on their personalities and their life situations. For example, if you are an active member of the military, your values or your security are not likely to come from having cash on hand. As a soldier you need to make money, but mostly your professional success is measured by how well you defend your country. If you work in the finance sector, where money (and lots of it) is the gauge for your sense of wealth and wellbeing and accomplishment, you are going to have a very different take on what constitutes "security."

You can be a billionaire who never needs to worry about money for the rest of your life, but if you are insecure about your health, all the houses and cars and safety deposit boxes don't mean much.

I see proof of this every day in my office. The rich and powerful men who need my attention to their health issues come with their (metaphorical) shields raised and armor on. They leave in a very different emotional state. One extremely well-known CEO with a particularly fearsome reputation started crying during one of our appointments. He was having a terrible time worrying about whether he had a serious, even lethal illness, and he had no one he could confide in. His tears were warranted.

"Did you ever see a CEO cry before?" he asked as he wiped his eyes.

"I see it all the time," I told him.

He smiled weakly, and I could see some of the tension leave his body. For once in his life, he was glad to share the spotlight, as it were. I couldn't tell him how many men like him had sat in that chair opposite me, many of them titans of industry on the outside and scared, sad, and lonely men in my office. If men like him were truly secure, they wouldn't be CEOs—because in their world, they can't show emotional weakness, even though they're often driven by "I'll show you!" insecurities.

You know the type—has to be on top, has to be acknowledged as powerful, has to win at all costs, has to be ruthless along the way. They're brilliant at their jobs but insecure about something important—friendships, family, health, hair, physical appearance—because all their energy has been directed toward work goals, not personal ones. Titans of industry are often emotionally stunted beneath their Masters of the Universe veneer.

Why did this super-powerful man let his guard down enough to become so emotional in such a short time? Because I made him feel secure in my office. He knew no one else in his life—not even his wife—would listen to him without judgment. It made me wonder if he had a satisfying sex life. He probably didn't. And that gets back to my point that true security isn't just about a lot of zeroes in the bank. It's about trust and openness. And he had none.

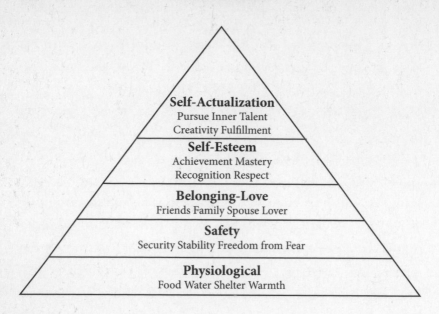

The Maslow Pyramid of Needs

Psychologist Abraham Maslow knew all about the need for trust and security. He developed a theory that he wrote about in a 1943 paper titled "A Theory of Human Motivation" (and later expanded into the book *Motivation and Personality*). Although he never used a pyramid himself to highlight his ideas, what he wrote about human needs struck such a nerve that it has become extremely well-known in pyramid form.

According to Maslow, human beings can only feel secure when their needs are met, and his hierarchy ranked these needs into five categories. At the bottom of the pyramid is the most fundamental security need, physical survival, followed by safety (these days, those would be personal and financial security, safety nets for hard times, and health and wellness security), and then belonging (to a community, to a family, and with a partner). After that comes self-esteem (which is where a career giving you satisfaction fits in) and finally self-actualization (being most yourself and your most creative) at the top.

It may be an older model, but it still resonates, and I use it with most of my patients. I know that if they aren't getting their basic needs met—and great sex certainly falls into this category!—they aren't going to feel secure. Some of them (usually high-powered titans of industry) look at me blankly when I mention that self-actualization is really about giving back, and that can only happen when you're feeling secure about all other aspects of your life. Women, on the other hand, usually get it right away.

I explain that you need to be grounded in the four bottom levels of needs before anything else can happen in your life. If you don't have a home or a good job, for example, you will need to expend all of your energy on finding one, and you won't have a lot of energy left over for other pursuits. Once you've established the basics, though, you can move up the pyramid.

Once you reach the top, you can not only develop your creative fulfillment, but also spend time giving back. Not just with money or time, but with everything you do. A person whose needs have been met and who is wholly secure is usually a person who wants to be giving, present, and loving for others.

This notion was proven by researchers at the University of Virginia, who conducted a study which involved more than 1,400 heterosexual couples between the ages of eighteen and forty-six. The researchers discovered that couples who reported a high level of generosity in their relationship—the amount of giving, whether emotional or shared chores or just taking care of the daily running of the household—were five times more likely to say they have a "very happy" marriage and a high level of sexual satisfaction.

"What happens outside of the bedroom seems to matter a great deal in predicting how happy husbands and wives are with what happens in the bedroom," noted W. Bradford Wilcox, associate professor of sociology at the University of Virginia and one of the study researchers.

Giving back pays forward in countless ways. It makes you feel better about yourself, which makes you happier, which makes you feel more secure about who you are, which gives you confidence, which makes you feel more attractive, which attracts like-minded people to you, which makes you even happier... Well, you see where I'm going with this!

So let me bring the need for security and this concept of generosity back to sex.

Five Infallible Rules for Sexual Security

You can ensure your sexual security—and your relationship happiness—by following these infallible rules.

Infallible Rule 1

- No judgments. Being judgmental is the kiss of death when you or your partner needs to feel secure. If you are critical of your loved ones, especially when they're feeling blue or vulnerable, they're less likely to open up, and their insecurities will deepen.

- You have to take risks, because opening up your heart makes you vulnerable. Falling in love is risky because you can get hurt. But you have to make yourself vulnerable to have a great relationship. Taking your clothes off and lying there naked in bed is awfully vulnerable, right? Even more so when you open up emotionally. But when you trust your partner and are secure in each other's love, the risks start to seem much less risky. The only way for this to happen is to take those risks in the first place.

Infallible Rule 2

- In the bedroom, make sure your partner is pleased first. When you both get into bed with that attitude, you'll be in perfect harmony because you'll both be striving for the same goal. You don't always have to be on top, but it's all right for you to take the lead once in a while.
- You might not have spontaneous orgasms, but that's not the point. The point is that if you always want to make your partner feel good first, he or she will know it and want to please you back. You will know he wants to do that, which will make you happy and relaxed. And then you have even better sex. It's a lot easier than you think!

Infallible Rule 3

- Be a good listener. You already learned how to do that in Lesson 5. Make sure your partner has his ears open, too!
- Acknowledge your partner's desires, and be certain he does the same. (You'll learn more about this in Lesson 7.)

Infallible Rule 4

- If you spend too much time worrying about what other people are thinking, you'll be so insecure about yourself that you won't be able to receive love as you are giving it. Most people aren't thinking what *you're* thinking about you! (Believe me, your partner is not thinking about the size of your thighs when you've got him all hot and bothered in bed.)

Infallible Rule 5

- Don't hold on to anger or frustration. If you go to bed nursing a grudge, you're not going to relax and enjoy having sex—and your partner is going to sense how you feel and respond with insecurity. Think of what British diplomat Harold Nicholson wisely said: "I think the secret of a successful marriage is the capacity to treat disasters as if they were incidents and not to magnify incidents into disasters." Try to live by those words, even when you want to throttle your partner!

The Gift of Security

One of the easiest ways to make people feel happy and secure is to bring a gift. If you're invited to a dinner party, you pick up a bottle of wine or some flowers to make your host feel happy and secure in the fact that you clearly want to be there. But you can give a host or hostess an even better gift, one that will improve your relationship and your sex life, too. And best of all, you don't need to spend any money on this gift of security.

What makes people feel secure is you giving them the gift of thoughtfulness:

Bring a compliment, a joke, a smile.
Bring positive energy.
Bring good manners and a polite demeanor, even if the people you're speaking to are mind-numbingly boring and rude.
Bring your energy to perk up the environment and the people in it.

I promise that once you start doing this, you will bring this attitude to bed with you, and it will rub off on your partner. (And your children. And colleagues. And friends.)

If you want to spend money on a special gift for a special someone, use the same thoughtfulness. Using LSD doesn't just have to be for your partner. I'll never forget how, one day, I was out shopping with a friend and we walked by one of those stores that sells gadgets you'd never think of but want when you see them. We went inside and I saw a funny-looking object that I realized was a shoe shiner—it rotated when you turned it on. I laughed and made some offhand remark about what a genius idea that was for someone like me who loved his shoes to be highly polished. My friend laughed, too.

Fast-forward to my birthday, ten months later. A big box arrived, and it was the shoe-shiner, along with a funny note.

This happened about twenty years ago, but I can still remember the swift pang of happiness I got when I opened that box. Not because my friend had spent a lot of money. Because he'd listened to me. He knew what my desire was. And getting such a crazy, thoughtful gift I never would have bought myself made me secure in my friendship with him.

Apply that to your relationship, and you've not only got a great partnership going on, but you're going to see some great improvements in your sex life, too. That's the essence of LSD!

Check Your Attitude at the Door

It can take only a few words to build up your sense of security, and just as many to break it down in a flash.

I was at a dinner in a restaurant once, and the man at the next table had a very loud and booming voice. He also had a very loud and booming attitude.

"I'm so good-looking," said this egomaniac, "that I can get any woman in this place to go to bed with me."

I'm not kidding. He really said that. Is a man like that ever going to make a woman feel secure? Of course not. These emotional characteristics are guaranteed security killers.

We all mess up when we don't really mean to, especially when we're with our partners. As I mentioned earlier, some of the most difficult feelings to manage are when we're:

- **Judgmental:** "You're wearing that?" "I can't believe you think that is so great. It really stinks."
- **Dismissive:** "Of course you wouldn't understand." "Whatever you say."
- **Superior:** "I started driving before you did, so don't tell me how to park." "I didn't think you knew that word."
- **Ego-driven:** "I know I'm the best at this." "She'll never be as smart as me."
- **Uncaring:** "So sorry, I have to be somewhere else." "It's not my problem that I'm always late."

Because it's only human nature to slip up, be aware if you have the tendency to act with any of these attitudes. Instead, strive to do the opposite, and be:

- **Nonjudgmental:** "I love the way you look." "I don't agree with your opinion, but I understand your reasons for it."
- **Embracing:** "You always have a distinctive spin on everything." "Tell me your ideas about this. I really want to know."
- **Supportive:** "You're a lot better at doing that than you think you are." "You're always there for me."
- **Ego-appropriate:** "I know I'm good at what I do because I've worked hard at it." "I do the best I can."
- **Caring:** "Tell me what you need. How can I help you?" "I really do love you."

Dear Dr. Fisch: His Insecurity about His Baldness Is Driving Me Crazy

Dear Dr. Fisch,

My husband is twenty-nine and losing his hair. It doesn't bother me at all and I keep telling him how sexy he still is, but he is very, very upset. He is insecure about it to the point where it's starting to drive a wedge between us. I'm wondering how I can feel secure in this marriage when he's getting so bent out of shape about his head. How can I convince him that I still love him and find him attractive, with or without his hair?

Signed, Shampoo Girl

Dear Shampoo Girl,

It's great that you are so supportive of your husband, regardless of how he looks, but it sounds like his baldness could be a bigger deal than you realize. Going bald is almost always due to whatever genes a man inherited, and it happens to all of us—even if we're desperate to stop it!—though at different rates and in different patterns. It affects us men more than we let on and far more than women realize.

Just so you know, the basic cause of balding is a buildup of a hormone called dihydrotestosterone (DHT). The more he has, the sooner he'll look like Yul Brynner in *The King and I*. Drugs called reductase inhibitors can block or inhibit DHT; they're found in prescription meds like Finasteride and Propecia. But they don't work for everyone.

It's important not to be dismissive of your husband's concerns. Because baldness can be such a touchy and sensitive subject for men, he's looking for extra support from you. Try gently telling him what this relationship really means to you. Make it clear that you're not after the physical aspect but the emotional contact.

Don't assume that he understands how you really feel. Most men think they need to be the most macho guy on this planet, and that hair is an outward manifestation of macho-ness. We both know this is kind of silly, but it's *his* kind of silly!

Hopefully, your husband will relax when you tell him how much you love him and what you really want from your life together—and that his hair has little to do with the big picture of your future. That should be enough to help him get past this tricky issue.

It's Hard to Feel Secure about Anything When You're Stressed

We all get stressed. It's part of life. But when you're super-stressed and exhausted, your sex life can suffer. Some people find that having lots of sex can help them manage their stress, because concentrating on giving and receiving pleasure can temporarily minimize other worries. Others find it impossible to relax or even be touched when they're stressed. If you want a lot of sex and your partner doesn't want any that could create even more stress. Clearly, some compromising is going to have to happen.

It's crucial that every couple incorporate stress-busters into their regular routine, together or separately. Find something you love—that makes you feel good and can help you relax or unwind—and do it. For me, that's playing tennis. Hitting the ball for hours helps the tension melt away. Indeed, exercise is one of the most effective stress-busters there is. Try working out on your own, or plan hikes or runs or bike rides together.

See if you can develop hobbies, too. I have friends who love to garden. They're both outside, working toward the common goal of making their garden more beautiful, but engaged in different tasks at the same time. The time is brilliantly well-spent where they're doing something they both adore, each in their own way.

Some people need to manage their stress on their own. They like to take long baths or go for solitary walks or play solitaire or read a book. You aren't being selfish if you need to take care of yourself! Everyone needs their own space so they can recharge their batteries. The less stress you have—and the more your partner encourages your stress-busting—the more likely you'll be in a relaxed and happy mood and ready for sex.

Security = Creating Your Own Nest

When Juliet called in to my radio show, I could immediately hear the frustration in her voice.

"My boyfriend is going to propose," she said, "and I know he got the ring already. But I don't want to marry him."

"Why don't you want to marry him? What kind of work does he do?" I asked. I had an intuitive flash about what her answer would be. There are many reasons not to want to get married, of course, but I had a feeling about what she was about to say.

"Oh, he's not working right now."

Boom! There you have it. He wasn't working, and Juliet was internally telling herself, "You know what? You can do better. You need someone who can take care of you the way you know you can take care of him."

Her boyfriend wasn't going to be able to help her live in the kind of nest she needed, so she wanted out.

One of my frequent tennis partners is in the same sort of situation. He's a highly paid, high-powered executive who'd been working all his life. But with the current economy, he lost his job a year ago and is really depressed. How is he dealing with this situation? By playing more tennis. Sure, it helps with his frustration and anxiety and gives him something to focus on, but his wife is ready to throttle him. She doesn't care if he plays a lot of tennis—but *only* after he's spent most of his time networking or pounding the pavement in search of work.

Not surprisingly, their sex life is nonexistent.

He's too stuck in frustration and depression to be able to perform, and she's too stuck in frustration and anger to have any desire for him.

From the gist of my conversation with Juliet, she clearly wasn't expecting her boyfriend to be a power player, and having a lot of money wasn't the most important factor in her getting married. Nor is my friend's frustrated wife going to kick him out of the house and demand a divorce. The point of these stories is not whether you have a good job or none at all. It's that you need to put in the *effort* to make your partner feel secure.

An analogy I like to use is about birds making their nests. Birds are biologically programmed to work together on a shared goal. Without a sturdy nest that took time and energy to build properly, that's safe from predators and lined with twigs and leaves and feathers so future generations can grow, the eggs won't be safe enough to hatch and thrive.

Similarly, you need the basic tools to make a nest for your family. That's where the enduring image of the white picket fence enclosing a home of your own comes from. People want security, so it's important for you as a couple to create a comfortable environment together that's your special haven. It doesn't have to be the bedroom—it can be the living room or even the kitchen, as long as it's a place that makes you feel secure.

This doesn't mean that you need an enormous amount of money to feel secure. What you need is confidence in your relationship so you can create your own safe haven together, one where you can shut the door to the outside world and feel secure in your love for each other in the nest you're building. That way, no matter what hits you in life, you have the strength of each other to see you through.

As long as you can talk openly about money and desire!

Is This You? Catching Your Patterns

Now that you have some strategies for bringing security into your relationship, take a look at these "he said, she said" conversations. They'll give you a good sense of what to watch out for.

Carter and Carolina: Out of the Fire and into a Rut

Carter is twenty-six and just out of the military. Despite his service, he's having trouble landing a full-time job in this economy, so he's been playing a lot of basketball with a semi-professional team. His wife, Carolina, knows how hard it is to find work, but she's still getting fed up. Although they've only been married for a few years and spent much of that time apart, she's already thinking about divorce.

Carter: I keep telling Carolina that playing basketball isn't just for fun. I hope I can make some money out of it.

Carolina: But that's not helping us now.

Carter: My friends on the team are going to help me.

Carolina: That's just a lot of talk. Nothing's come of it.

Their pattern: Carolina made her need for her nest very clear. She's worried about money. Carter seems a bit lost since he got out of the military, and he's avoiding the issue of finding work by hoping someone on his team will help him out.

My advice: Carter needs to understand how important it is for his wife to feel secure in their home and in the future they are going to create together. She needs to see concrete action from him that shows he can provide for her. That's the only way she'll be able to respect and trust him.

I understand that he's putting all his energy into playing basketball in hope that this will turn into a career someday, but frankly those dreams are unrealistic and, at this stage in his life, quite impractical. It's time for him to grow up and move on. He has a wife and a marriage and more responsibilities. Even if nothing comes his way at first, he needs to make the effort and start pounding the pavement.

First, he should sit down and strategize with Carolina about where to look and what kind of jobs might suit him. Perhaps, for example, he could use his physical prowess to become an athletic coach or trainer. He could see if there are courses he can take to become accredited and certified.

Once Carolina sees how serious he is about looking for work, she will stop threatening to leave. As soon as Carter gets work, he will be providing for them financially, and he'll be making her feel a lot happier in their relationship.

Donnie and Kara: Keep the Kids in the Classroom

Donnie's fiancée is a kindergarten teacher, and she can't seem to leave the classroom behind when she leaves work. She tends to treat Donnie like one of her students, and he feels diminished, patronized, and insecure about his role as the adult male in their relationship. (This may sound familiar—we looked at a similar example earlier with Connor and Emily.)

Kara doesn't think she's doing anything wrong, but Donnie is having trouble reaching orgasm during sex, mainly because he masturbates so much because it gives him some measure of control. Kara has no idea how much self-stimulation goes on when she's out of the house or asleep.

> **Donnie**: I really hate it when you talk to me like a five-year-old.
> **Kara**: I don't know what you're talking about.
> **Donnie**: Yes, you do. You're always telling me what to do in that singsongy voice you use with the kids. You're always correcting me. Even when we're having sex.
> **Kara**: I am?

Their pattern: Kara has no idea how emasculated Donnie feels because he thinks she treats him like a kid. She tells him what to do and he does it, but until now, he hasn't spoken up about his frustration and insecurity.

My advice: This is a couple that has real problems communicating. Until now, Donnie hasn't been able to voice his feelings, and this has created a big issue for them in the bedroom. He can't take the initiative because Kara is always telling him what to do, and she is completely unaware of what's going on.

To make matters worse, Donnie has become a chronic masturbator, which makes it difficult for him to be aroused by Kara. This is a classic example of retarded ejaculation, and it's a dangerous path for their relationship.

None of this is a good sign for their upcoming marriage. Donnie needs to man up and tell Kara how he feels. She's not a mind reader, and if she thought their sex life was fine when it wasn't, she has to be told. They need to clear some time and have a long, honest talk about what needs to change to make things work. They should make a five-things list, each writing down five things they love about each other and the five things they'd like to change.

Donnie's list should include how he feels when Kara treats him like a kindergarten student. In addition, as embarrassing as this might be, he need to tell her about his masturbation habit. That's the kind of secret that can end a relationship, especially for a couple planning a life together. By dealing with these issues now, they can start their marriage on a trusting note of honesty and openness about sharing, which should serve them well over their lifetime together. Kara will be able to keep her teaching in the classroom, and Donnie will feel stronger in his masculinity and his ability to make her happy in bed.

Michael and Emily: The Thirty-Year Itch

Michael and Emily have been married for nearly thirty years, and their children are grown and out of the house. Emily is going through menopause and is having a tough time. She's gained a lot of weight, and that embarrasses her. Worse, she's not interested in sex, even saying that it hurts, and it's tearing her marriage apart.

Michael has gotten so frustrated that he cheated on Emily several times. He still loves Emily very much and knows that her avoidance of sex is no excuse for having affairs. He feels deeply contrite and wants to repair their marriage. But he doesn't know if that's possible when Emily refuses to have sex.

> **Emily**: I know Michael didn't mean to hurt me. It's all my fault.
> **Michael**: No, it isn't. I still love you and shouldn't have given in to temptation. But you won't have sex with me—you won't even let me see you after you take a shower. I mean, come on. We've been married for thirty years already. I don't care if you've put on a few pounds.
> **Emily**: But I do. I'm trying, really, I am. And I still love you, too. I just don't care about sex anymore. It doesn't feel good and I don't want to do it.
> **Michael**: Do you honestly expect me to spend the rest of my life not having any sex?
> **Emily**: No. I don't know what to do.

Their pattern: This is a tough situation. They clearly care about each other deeply, but they're at an impasse. Emily is stuck in denial and incapable of compromise. Michael wants to do the right thing but is suffering from severe sexual (and emotional) frustration. They have the same conversation over and over, but unless Emily deals with her issues, she's going to keep pushing Michael away—and she knows it.

My advice: Michael and Emily are being tested in every way possible. This marriage has hit a rough patch, one that is common for couples when physical changes create emotional changes.

Emily needs to have a thorough checkup with her gynecologist to explore whether any physical reasons would explain why sex is no longer enjoyable for her, and especially why it hurts her. Her hormonal levels have dropped considerably, and she might be a candidate for hormone replacement therapy that could improve her libido. Or, it's possible that she has a bladder that has prolapsed (fallen out of its normal position).

Most of all, she needs to be told by her gynecologist that many, if not most, women are able to maintain an active sex life while going through menopause. It may require some adjustments, such as using a good-quality lubricant or finding sexual positions that allow women to be more fully satisfied.

She should also find a fitness program, including strength training that will help her lose weight, tone her muscles, and feel better about her body. The changes she's undergone are not uncommon. But Emily can't fix her sex life if she remains stuck in denial about her physical and emotional health.

Michael needs to acknowledge how painful his affairs have been for Emily, even if she's blaming herself. Her doing that is clear evidence of how full-blown her insecurities are. There's a real issue of trust, and he will help Emily greatly if he promises to be faithful while they both work through this hard time. If what he really wants is to have sex more often with her, he'll need to be patient and stand by her while she takes the steps she needs to get better. This may take a lot of time and love, and he needs to decide if he's willing to be there for her (and be temporarily sexually frustrated) or not.

Fortunately, they clearly still love each other very much, but restoring intimacy in this context is going to take a major effort at communication. I think they would hugely benefit from seeing a couples' therapist who could help them both better understand each other and the barriers that may exist to physical and emotional closeness.

The fact that they haven't divorced each other after thirty years together tells me that they both want to hang on. I firmly believe that they can work this out, but it's not going to be easy. Ideally, they'll find a solution to the sex issue that will be satisfying for both, and they'll be able to look back on this period as the challenging time that, ultimately, brought them closer together.

You Need a Date Night, But How Can You Go Out and Have Fun When You're on a Tight Budget?

Sometimes you have to get out of your nest to feel secure. Vacations are crucial whenever possible, because getting out of familiar surroundings can help you decompress. Vacations don't need to be expensive—you can stay in a motel a few hours' drive away. The point is leaving your daily life behind for a short while so you can spend time with the person you love most. That strengthens your bond and makes your partner feel secure.

Vacations don't happen often for most people, but you still need to find time to be alone with your partner, where you can talk without distractions about everything that's important or not important or just fun. Studies have shown that couples who have regular date nights are much more likely to have a great sexual relationship. They're showing each other how important it is to clear their calendars so they can be together. Away from work. Away from the kids.

And away from all digital devices that intrude on your intimate moments!

If you're on a tight budget, as most people are, you can still have date night without breaking the bank. Use cash only wherever you can so you don't overspend. Look for nearby restaurants that have regular deals or discounts, and go online to find coupons or special offers. Find a cheap and cheerful place that becomes your "local." Once you're a regular, you'll likely notice freebies coming your way from the owner who appreciates repeat business.

Go on a picnic and bring some great food you made yourself. Put all your loose change into the date-night jar, and when you have enough, splurge on tickets to a sporting event or a movie you both want to see. If you live in or near a city, there are always free things to do that can often be more enjoyable than big-ticket events.

A little date-night effort and imagination will go a long way toward keeping couples working in sync with each other. Feeling safe, feeling loved, and feeling secure.

LESSON 7

D IS FOR DESIRE
...YOU'VE GOT TO SHOW IT TO KNOW IT

Desire is such an evocative word. It makes me think of all the things I desire: the touch of my wife's hand, the sound of my children's laughter, good health, a chocolate-covered donut, a fierce tennis game (that I win), my friendships, and the satisfaction of knowing I am helping my patients.

And desire in bed, too, of course. For me, sexual desire is all about making sure that both of us are satisfied.

More than that, desire isn't just about a sexual craving for your lover, about his kisses and his hands on your skin and your time in bed together. It means you care about your partner—and that you demonstrably *show* that you care.

"Would it kill you to be nice?" one of my friends' moms used to say to us when we were little kids horsing around. She drove me crazy at the time, but there's a lot of wisdom in those words. It's so much easier to show your desire for your partner, to be nice, than to be nasty or forgetful, or to take someone you love for granted.

Let me give you a rather blunt example from a couple who called in to my radio show.

"She never wants to have sex with me anymore! We've only been married for five years, and it's not right, I tell ya. It's not fair. It doesn't matter what I say to her. I'm going crazy," said the husband.

"Let me hear what your wife has to say," I told him. As I've said before, if a man isn't getting any sex, there's always a valid reason.

"I'll tell you why he isn't getting any," said his wife as soon as she got on the air. "Do you know how fat and disgusting he is?" she asked. "He's like a hundred pounds overweight, never takes a shower, doesn't care what he looks like, doesn't care about his health, doesn't care how worried I am about him, nothing. So he has some nerve complaining about me not having sex with him when he's a big, fat, stinking slob. *And I am not going to bed with a man who's a slob!*"

The husband got very silent. Then he hung up.

Really, what could he say to that—except maybe, "I'm so sorry, honey. I'm going to start taking better care of myself, not just for you, but for me. And I'm jumping in the shower right now."

But clearly he wasn't ready to say that.

The verdict on this marriage: doomed to fall into the recrimination trap (which can look a lot like quicksand) unless he does the work to make his wife desire him. His slovenly ways made him so physically unappealing that his wife's libido took an understandable plunge. And he realizes that just because he desires *her* doesn't mean he deserves her desire in return.

Dear Dr. Fisch: My Wife Had Breast Implants and I'm Scared

Dear Dr. Fisch,

For as long as I've known her, my wife (we've been married for three years) has been obsessed with how small her breasts are. I really liked them, and it didn't bother me at all. But she saved up her money and went from an A cup to a C cup. I like her new breasts, too, but I'm worried that she's cheating on me. What should I do?

Signed, Feeling Like a Booby

Dear Feeling Like a Booby,

The question you need to have answered is: Does my wife want sexual attention and to be desired by other men, or is she just empowering her ability to change what she wants to change? The answer might be right in front of you. If your wife is wearing the same kind of clothes but just has a bigger cup size, I wouldn't worry. An A cup is small for most women, and if enlarging her breasts was something she thought through carefully and decided would make her happy, then more power to her. But if she's now wearing provocative clothing that flaunts her cleavage, that's a different story.

My advice is to acknowledge and praise her determination to act on a desire that was important for her and to give her the attention—your attention as her husband—that tells her, yes, you have a lovely new body and I love it because it's yours. Buy her some sexy lingerie that will showcase her breasts, and she'll be thrilled. It's thoughtful, and ironically your willingness to go with the flow on this one will show her that you will love and value her regardless of what she looks like.

Remember, just because a woman changes the size of her breasts doesn't mean she's changing anything else, especially the way she feels about you. Inside, she's still the same woman you love.

How to Express Your Desires

I've seen so many couples in my office that I've become good at placing them on the "How Much We Desire Each Other" scale. I'm not being glib about this, because most of these couples are enduring a stressful situation. They might be suffering from infertility and desperate to have a baby. The woman might be more desperate for this baby than the husband. Or perhaps he's affected by a medical condition, such as a serious type of sexual dysfunction.

Tipping the scales into perfect balance are couples who are stressed yet who still desire each other. They show this in subtle yet telling ways. They sit close to each other. They hold hands, not just because they're nervous, but because they want to touch the other. They look at each other when one of them is talking, or they finish each other's sentences, not because one is interrupting, but because they're so good at knowing what he or she is going to say. They smile and nod and murmur words of encouragement. They're in sync.

So whatever their problem is, I know they'll work with me as a team to get it fixed.

A couple stuck at a lower end of the "Desire Each Other" scale shows it, too. They fold their arms. They don't look at each other, or if they do, it's with frustration or anger. The man often looks out the window or sneaks peeks at his cell phone. They interrupt each other. They pick a fight. Their scale is tipping so badly to one side that it's nearly broken. They're in trouble, and I know it.

What I tell these couples is that, if they're committed to making their relationship work, they need to become better at expressing their needs.

And they need to start with LSD. Listening and feeling secure, which will lead to desire.

With it, they can find happiness again. Without it, their future as a couple is at risk.

You've Got to Show It to Know It

When was the last time you told your partner how much you desired him or her? Not just "I love you" or "I like you" or "Thank you for picking the kids up from soccer practice."

I mean, when was the last time you called your partner and said, "Honey, I can't wait 'til the kids go to bed tonight because all I want is to be with you"? Something original and different.

If you're like most couples who are stuck in a rut, it's been a long time since this desire was openly expressed. Yet adding desire into your daily routine is simple to do. And a little bit goes a long way toward making your partner not only happy and secure, but flooded with desire for you, too.

Here's what to do:

Make Your Desires Clear

Even when you know what you want to say, it's often difficult to say it, especially if you're not sure about the reaction. I've found that it's much easier to communicate when you write things down.

Just as you did with the "I Need Five Things during Sex" list, follow these steps and create a new "Five Things I Desire" list. (This strategy is so effective that it's worth using for any similar situation.)

- Get a pad of paper and a pen or pencil. Again, don't type on a keyboard—*write*. The personal act of writing will make you feel more invested in this list, which in turn will make you more likely to act on it. (Hello, better relationship and better sex!)
- Draw a line down the middle.
- At the top of the left-side column, write "What I Love about You."
- At the top of the right-side column, write "What I Desire from You." (Or "What I'd Like You to Do to Me in Bed." Tweak it as needed.)
- List as least three things in each column. Five is better.
- Be clear in your mind exactly what you want to communicate with your partner. This way, you're being completely honest about your desires and reinforcing them with what you love about him, too.
- Be as brief and concrete as possible. That means using as few words as you can to still make your point. Men tune out quickly, so if you're not specific, they're not going to get it.
- Ask your partner to do his own list.

- Read each other's lists in an environment where you won't be interrupted. I always tell my patients to go out to dinner and do this. You'll be in a relaxed environment away from your regular stresses.

Or sometimes I have couples do this in my office. I've never seen it fail.

"Oh, you feel that way about me?" is what I'll hear.

Or, "You really want that? I had no idea!"

When I hear that, I know there's going to be a lot of great sex that night!

Act on Your Desires—and Have Him Act on His

Now that you've made your desires clear, it's time to act on them. For example:

- First thing to do in the morning, whisper some sweet nothing in your partner's ear.
- Write notes on Post its and stash them in secret places in your partner's briefcase, lunch bag, purse—whatever they bring to work—to give them a little naughty surprise. (Make sure your notes aren't not too revealing, in case someone at work spies them!)
- Text your partner during the day. Say, "Thinking of you," or "Love you," or "Can't wait to get home" or "See you soon." Use emoticons that you know make your partner laugh.
- Don't expect replies.
- Send a private tweet. (It's short, so you don't have to be clever.)
- Pick up the phone, say something sweet, and hang up.

- Make a random compliment about something you never compliment. (Just be sincere!)

Believe me, your partner will get the message very quickly. Then he will start taking the lead.

What's so brilliant about this kind of desire-making is how little effort it takes. I mean, really little. A few seconds of time will reap hours of pleasure in bed later.

Just remember that there's a fine line between showing your partner how much you are thinking about him or her, and your partner thinking you are overdoing it for some reason. Have fun with this, but don't go too crazy, especially if your partner is having a busy time at work.

Once you and your partner get into the habit of acknowledging your love and desire for each other—because that's what this is all about, after all—you will find yourself doing this to all those who are important in your orbit. It's a great habit to have for life.

Spice Up Your Sex Life (within Limits!)

Acting on your desires is only part of what keeps couples happy. You need to ensure that this desire is always fresh and fun. Sometimes you'll crave the comfortable, tried-and-true sexual behavior that you know brings forth satisfying orgasms. And sometimes, you'll want to spice things up by getting inventive.

Joe and his wife, Alice, came to see me. I could tell Alice was not happy. On the "How Much We Desire Each Other" scale, the tipping-off point was about to be reached. Their once-robust sex life had dwindled to practically nothing, and when they did make love, Joe made demands that Alice didn't like.

"All he wants to do is watch pornography, and he treats me like his own personal porn star who's supposed to do whatever he says and *love* it," she told me as they both sat in my office.

"So how do we get around that?" I asked. "One simple word: *Compromise*."

Alice and Joe looked at each other warily.

"Joe, let me ask you. What would you like to watch?" I said. "What would please you the most?

"Well, maybe she could dress up a little bit," he said.

"All right, Alice, is that okay?" I asked.

"Yes. I could dress up."

"You *would*?" Joe practically keeled over in shock. He'd never thought to ask!

"Well, what do you want to dress up in?" I continued. "How about a nurse's outfit?"

"Oh, I could do that," Alice said, a coy smile teasing at the corner of her lips. "In fact, I can do one better. It'll be a nice surprise."

As you can imagine, Joe was practically salivating. With a little bit of honest communication and openness, he was able to have one of his fantasies come to life, and Alice was able to participate in a way that made her comfortable. I knew there would be no porn watching in their house later that night!

See how a little bit of LSD works? A little bit of listening. Exploration of needs and wants in a safe and calm way that made Alice and Joe feel secure. And a clear acknowledgment that a bit of compromise could increase their desire for each other.

This is one of the most common scenarios I deal with. The woman tells me that her husband doesn't desire her anymore and doesn't want to have sex with her. Then I ask the man what he wants his partner to do. He tells me he'd love it if she could just dress up a little bit or another relatively simple request.

And then what do the women do? They almost always say, "I'd love to do that. *But he never asked me to do that before.*"

As we've seen before, what Alice and Joe and other couples mentioned in this book had trouble understanding was how fantasies play an important role in sex. Fantasies are normal. They allow couples to invent scenarios in their heads and act on them, which keeps the sex fresh. By allowing your flights of fancy to happen, you can turn even the same old, same old into a thrilling adventure. Finding ways to add variety to your sex life is a much better solution than seeking the "spice" outside the relationship.

Dear Dr. Fisch: Keeping Our Sex Life Spicy

Dear Dr. Fisch,

My husband, Francisco, and I have been married for seventeen years and we have seven kids. We have a great sex life, sometimes having sex two or three times a day, and like to try new things. Sometimes we even download or rent porn and watch it together, sometimes before we have sex and sometimes during. We like to try new positions and do lots of role-playing, but I draw the line at more hardcore or kinky stuff. What else can we do to spice up our sex life?

Signed, Can't Help Loving That Man of Mine

Dear Can't Help Loving That Man of Mine,

You sound like a very sexually healthy couple to me. The fact that you occasionally watch porn together is totally fine. What you're watching isn't a necessity for you to get aroused, so you're not relying on it. It's like porn is your dessert—sometimes you want to indulge in, and most of the time you can live without it.

I have to say that if you're having sex two or three times a day, I am in awe! That's way above average, especially with seven kids. Wondering if your sex life will get boring can be an issue in any long-term relationship, but I honestly think you two are doing all the right things.

All I can advise you to do is continue doing what you're doing. There are lots of different positions you can try, and keep on being inventive. It's always a turn-on for partners to be endlessly inventive and willing. As long as you're communicating openly with each other, and your occasional porn viewing and sex play is helping and not harming your sex life, I don't see any problem in your relationship.

Just make sure to keep the bedroom door locked so the kids don't get in!

Fifty Shades of Fantasies: What Women Want from Men (and Might Not Want to Tell Them)

Did you know that one of the most common female fantasies is to be "taken"? Not hurt, certainly not raped, but *ravished*. That's the note that runs through romance novels. It has also fueled the *Fifty Shades of Grey* erotica that has, interestingly enough, made it more okay for women to talk candidly about their fantasies and the fact that they might like to role-play as submissive or dominant in bed.

In other words, what some women want (at least some of the time) is for a man to really take charge during sex. To be confident, to be demanding (without being a bully), to not fumble. A man who isn't afraid to take an active role and to tumble on the bed.

What's important to understand here is that role-playing during sex has nothing to do with your roles as partners, parents, or professionals outside the bedroom. This is what constantly trips people up. They think that they have to be the same during sex as they are during the day.

If you want great sex, it's time to get out of your comfort zone and have some fun! Push some boundaries and discover your edge. Trusting your partner to help you live out your fantasies is a brilliant way to reinforce how secure you feel with each other.

And realize this: you might be equals in every way, but in the bedroom, someone always has to be on top. One day it can be you, and the next day it can be your partner. However you work it out, if you're always trying to be all sweet and fair in bed, time after time, your sex life is going to get very boring very quickly.

If you want great sex for life, you need to see it as a great adventure. You never know where the road is going to lead you. This list will show you how.

How to Safely Express Your Fantasies

First, make sure you know exactly what you want to communicate with him before you get started. Men need to hear your desires in very concrete terms, or chances are they're not going to know what they need to do to help you.

1. Make Your Fantasies Clear

As you did in making your desires clear, it's helpful to make a fantasies list. Follow the steps on page 238—with one big caveat: If you ask your partner to share his fantasies with you, you can't make any judgments. Even if your initial reaction is shock (or disgust), you are asking your partner to share his innermost thoughts with you. This is not the time to be judgmental.

If you make a face or say, "Oh my God, you want to wear my silk panties? That's just *disgusting*!" he's definitely not going to want to share other fantasies with you in the future, and he certainly won't want to help spice up your sex life further. (Fantasies come in all shapes and sizes; one of the most common fantasies I hear from men is they want their partner to dress up in… bike shorts.) So be prepared in advance to handle your partner's fantasy list.

You also don't have to agree to everything that's suggested! Remember, these are *fantasies*. Having them doesn't always mean that they can or should be acted upon. If you find your partner's fantasy truly repellent, try not to be critical or react with disgust. Simply say, "I don't want to that and I will not do that. But maybe we could do this instead."

For example, a common male fantasy is to have a threesome, with you being one of the two women in bed with him. Don't worry that this means your husband wants to cheat on you, and don't see it as negative. It just means that he trusts you enough to confide that this is one of his fantasies, and he wants to include you in them. It does *not* mean you need to have a threesome or that he needs to, either.

2. Role Playing and Acting Out Your Fantasies

Now that you both have made your desires and fantasies clearer, it's time to have some fun. A few tips:

- Go into this with an open mind. If you think you're going to have fun, you will.
- Be playful. Be creative. Laugh a lot.
- Make rules about what can or can't be done. It's all about compromise.
- As I discussed in Lesson 6, the best way to have great sex is to go into the bedroom trying to make your partner be happier than you are. It'll never work if one partner says, "*Service* me now" and that's not part of the agreed-upon role-playing. I think that's one of the reasons why women get so fed up by men who want oral sex. So few men offer to return the favor that women can feel like they're only there to service their partner's needs. Let me tell you, guys, that is a major turnoff.
- If your partner is hesitant, start with small changes—trying a new position, for example. Don't leap right into anal sex or bondage.
- If acting out your fantasy isn't quite as much fun as what you fantasized about, communicate effectively so that both of you can find a middle ground that makes the experience pleasurable.
- If one party demands that his or her fantasies be indulged

and the other party doesn't feel comfortable, that's not great sex. That's more like coercion!

3. Think about Props and Sex Toys (or Not!)

As you know by now, I am not a fan of vibrators, dildos, and other sex toys. When you use props a lot, you can get used to the props. That makes it harder to have sex without them.

I know that a lot of people—including sex therapists and many of my patients and radio callers—strongly disagree with me. That's fine. Taking a trip to a sex store to see toys that come in every possible shape, size, color, and texture—something for everyone!—can be an undeniable hoot for couples and certainly a bonding experience.

Some people even see these jaunts as a safe way to be able to express their fantasies. After all, seeing so much apparatus and stuff in these stores makes it far more normal to admit that you want to add some of these items to your sex play. Just be aware that sex without props or toys—just the two of you pleasuring each other—is, in my professional opinion, the best intimate experience.

4. Keep the Computers and Devices Out of the Bedroom

I've heard from many women that their partners are addicted to playing online games, and it's hurting their relationships. The choice should be a no-brainer, but these women rightly feel that their partners have more desire for virtual people and virtual games than for the real woman.

Research backs up this frustration. A study from Brigham Young University, published in the *Journal of Leisure Research,* found that 75 percent of the spouses of those who regularly play fantasy role-playing games, like World of Warcraft, wish their partner would spend less time gaming and more time on their marriage. The researchers found that it wasn't the game-playing itself that caused problems, but the arguing about it and the disrupted bedtime routines. In other words, the more someone was addicted to playing games, the less time he or she spent in bed having sex, great or otherwise. Clearly, his or her partner wouldn't be too happy about that.

If this is happening to you, there are two different strategies to try. The first is to set firm limits on game-playing with your spouse, just as you would with a child. The games need to be turned off by a specific time, for instance, or there will be consequences. This can be tough to do for those who are addicted. If so, the addict might need counseling or to go cold turkey, as addicts usually can't manage or kick their addictions on their own.

Another strategy is to find a game that you can play together. A game that hopefully will not have the same sort of addictive qualities. The gaming study I just mentioned also found that for couples in which both spouses play, 76 percent said that gaming led to higher marital satisfaction. I think that's because they were spending intense time together, doing something they both loved. It gave them goals and something fun to do and talk about. Some games can even inspire fantasies and role-playing.

Dear Dr. Fisch: My Fiancée Is Way Too Aggressive in Bed

Dear Dr. Fisch,

I've got a crazy problem. My fiancée always has to be in control when we're in bed. She told me the reason is that her last boyfriend before me was really aggressive and she had to be more submissive and she didn't like it. That wasn't the kind of sex that really pleases her. So, fine.

I kinda don't mind her being bossy because mostly it's fun, but lately she's been taking things too far. I woke up in the middle of the night and realized that she was fondling me in my sleep. I went nuts. She was taking total advantage of me, right? It wasn't fun—it was scary. I'm wondering what else she might be planning. How can I get her to take things down a notch?

Signed, Not in Control

Dear Not in Control,

You need to find a way to tell your fiancée that you're not comfortable with her level of aggressiveness without pushing her away. You realized that her touching you in your sleep is crossing a boundary that shouldn't be crossed. I understand that you're in love and planning your life together, but to make sure you stay on the right path, you need to screw up your courage and talk to her honestly about what goes on in bed. Do it now—or you'll be having more problems once you're married.

Perhaps because she was so submissive in her last relationship, she's overcompensating now. I suspect she really wants you to get a bit more aggressive yourself instead of giving in to her demands. Clearly, there's a happy middle ground somewhere where she can satisfy her need to be submissive or aggressive, while you change things up, too. In other words, she's acting like this to provoke you into becoming more aggressive and take control. This is why it's gotten more and more dangerous in bed. The longer she doesn't get what she wants, the more she's going to turn up the temperature between the sheets.

This is why you need to talk out precisely what you like to do and how much, and what's okay to explore and what's off-limits. Use the "Five Things I Desire" list from earlier in this lesson (see page 238) to spell out what you want. Next time you come home, tell her exactly how things are going to go down in the bedroom. She'll respect you for that, get turned on, and probably enjoy that you're taking charge.

If this doesn't work and you still don't feel comfortable with her bedroom behavior, she may not be the right person for you. Better to find out how sexually compatible you are before you get married than to go through a divorce because neither of you knew how to bring up the issue.

Is This You? Catching Your Patterns

Now that you have some strategies for bringing desire into your relationship, take a look at these "he said, she said" conversations. If these couples remind you of yourself and your partner, try my advice to make your relationship stronger.

Tommy and Elaine: Marriage Is Not a One-Way Street

Tommy and Elaine are both twenty-nine and have been married for three years. They didn't have much of a sexual relationship before they were married, and it's not going well now. The reason is simple: Tommy doesn't know much about what a marriage really means. He is so intent on getting his own needs met that their sexual relationship is completely lopsided. Elaine feels used and frustrated especially because the sex is over so quickly that she rarely has an orgasm.

> **Tommy**: I work hard all day, and I want to be serviced as soon as I get home.
>
> **Elaine**: You hear that? He said *serviced*. I'm not a freaking car!
>
> **Tommy**: Oh come on, you know what I mean. I just want to have sex when I want to have sex. That's why I got married.
>
> **Elaine**: You're crazy. I'm not your slave.
>
> **Tommy**: I never said you were. I don't know what you're talking about.
>
> **Elaine**: It's just about what you want. What about me?

Their pattern: Tommy is extremely immature about relationships—so clueless, obviously, that he thought he was marrying a sex slave. He just wanted sex without any emotional contact—and felt entitled to it. He thought by pouncing on Elaine as soon as he walked in the door, he was making his desire clear. He is in desperate need of sex education and relationship education to explain what being part of a couple means. He's so fixated on getting his desire met that he doesn't realize that his wife is entitled to her own desires, too.

My advice: First off, Tommy needs to understand that marriage isn't just about showing up and demanding sex. It's about growing together and maintaining an emotional connection. Elaine needed to find a way to tell Tommy to slow down in bed and to help him open up emotionally so they can strengthen their love for each other. I asked her what she wanted Tommy to do in bed, and to be very specific.

Elaine: It's not about him. I want more foreplay.
Tommy: What did you just say?
Elaine: Foreplay. You know. You get home and you kiss me for about thirty seconds, and then you're all ready to go. I need you to get down there and help me out for a few minutes because you know it takes me longer.
Tommy: Really?
Elaine: Yes, really.
Tommy: Oh, I didn't know that's what you wanted.

When I heard that, I explained that foreplay is crucial for women, but it isn't just about sexual stimulation. It's about making your partner feel loved and cared about. "I want you to put the dishes in the dishwasher or do some other chores around the house that you know Elaine doesn't like to do," I told Tommy.

"I want you to show her how much you care. Text her during the day. Ask if she wants a little drink before sex. Give her a massage first, before you've taken all your clothes off. Ask her what she wants you to do. Allow her to guide your fingers. And realize that sex is not going to be a two-minute sprint to the finish line anymore. Have fun together. Try lots of new positions. Take your time and really learn how to enjoy each other's bodies."

Tommy's eyes lit up when he heard this, and Elaine blushed and smiled. I wondered if Tommy would be able to expand his sexual repertoire from wham-bam to expert, and was gratified to find out that he quickly learned how to slow down, to become a better lover, and to make Elaine feel valued and cherished. In other words, he grew up once he changed his notions of what marriage meant and became a true partner to his wife.

Lewis and Carmen: Rekindling the Spark

Lewis and Carmen have been married for eight years and have two young children. He's thirty-nine and she's thirty-five. They both love each other deeply, but something is shifting in their marriage, which they regard as strong and committed and for life. What's shifted is the frequency and urgency of their sex life.

They had sex as often as five to six times a week when they were engaged and during their first year as a married couple, but it's gradually been diminishing to something that's more routine than exciting. It bothers them both. But they admit that they never talked about their sexual needs or desires when they were courting, or even after the wedding. They just did it. They need to get the spark and desire back into their sex life, pronto.

Lewis: My emotional connection to sex has diminished. So has how often we do it.

Carmen: I noticed it, too, starting around our first wedding anniversary.

Lewis: We weren't as spontaneous.

Carmen: I didn't want to have it as much, either.

Lewis: Then she got pregnant, and her morning sickness was so bad that our sex life practically disappeared.

Carmen: And when the baby was born, we were so tired we didn't think about it.

Lewis: Yeah, and nothing much changed after we had the second baby.

Carmen: So here we are.

Lewis: For me, it's more like a biological urge that needs to be taken care of, and for women it's much more connected to their emotions.

Carmen: Sometimes I feel that Lewis just wants to do it and get it over with, so he forgets to connect with me first. That just makes me feel like he's not interested in me or my body or my needs.

Their pattern: Like many married couples, what was once a wholly satisfying sex life has dwindled to infrequent forays that leave both partners dissatisfied and frustrated. But instead of talking frankly to each other, Lewis and Carmen remained silent. Their love was clear, but their communication skills were not.

My advice: I can tell they have a strong and loving marriage because they literally finish each other's thoughts. They might be having a rough patch sexually, but they are in complete emotional sync, and that is a terrific sign for them being able to work this out. Also, they both know that sexual intimacy is one of the most important aspects of a healthy sexual relationship. So is being able to express their sexual needs and desires, and that's what's tripping them up right now.

What I suggest they both do is be honest about what they want sexually. Use the "Five Things I Desire" list on page 238 to tell each other what they love about each other—and what they'd like to do and have done to each other. They can compare notes and take it from there. A certain amount of compromising might be needed at first—if, for example, Lewis wants sex four times a week and Carmen wants it less while they're working things through, perhaps they can settle on twice a week—but they should be able to come up with a mutually satisfying solution.

Then they can start using the suggestions in the "Act on Your Desires" list earlier in this lesson, on page 239. That ought to up the desire level on a daily basis.

Lewis and Carmen also need to realize that talking frankly about sex and your sexual needs is completely normal and healthy. They learned the hard way that even if you had a lot of sex when you were dating or in the first year of your marriage, if you don't make a conscious effort to discuss sex when you can, it almost becomes a taboo topic. And then the act becomes taboo in the bedroom. That's the last thing you want it to be!

Finally, they should try to set up date nights and only cancel them for true emergencies. I know how hard it can be to get out of the house when a couple has small children, but they need alone time as a couple to re-energize their desire for each other. I have no doubt that Carmen and Lewis's palpable love for each other will only get stronger as their intimacy deepens and they rediscover how much satisfying fun it is to have a great sex life.

Dear Dr. Fisch: My Girlfriend's a Dominatrix

Dear Dr. Fisch,

I'm forty-seven and my girlfriend, Vicky, is nineteen. She wants to be a model or an actress, and she has a smoking hot body if I do say so. We just moved and I'm having trouble finding work, so I'm depressed and frustrated. It's hard to get motivated. Vicky has a lot more energy, I have to say, and she's working as a dominatrix so we can make ends meet. Sometimes we get into some heavy kinds of drugs, especially during sex. Vicky is starting to tell me she loves me, but she's worried that this relationship is too wild to last. What do you think?

Signed, Getting Out of Control

Dear Getting Out of Control,

I hate to be blunt, but Vicky is right. I'm worried that there is a fundamental incompatibility here, and not only because of the age difference. Vicky is employed as a dominatrix, which makes her a professional sex worker in the kink-fetish community. Being a dominatrix doesn't involve having actual sex with her clients, but it's not a healthy profession, and obviously you're not feeling comfortable with it, either. She should be focusing on what both of you want to be doing with the rest of your lives.

If she is serious about acting and modeling, she should take classes and go on auditions and pursue those dreams, instead of expending her energy on unhealthy habits. I'm sure she wants a better life—and you want a better life for her. So do I. But I'll bet her comments to you are an indication that she's pretty much given up on having a future together with you.

It's also way past time for you to address your issues directly, especially your depression. Taking drugs is no way to deal with feelings of inadequacy and unhappiness, and will only lead to more serious problems down the road. All that does is help you avoid dealing with what you know needs to be dealt with, or worse (like ruining your health or getting you arrested).

It's vital that you focus now on getting a job and getting out of the house to lift your spirits and give you some clarity and direction in your life. I also recommend you explore why you feel you need to have a sexual relationship with someone who is so much younger than you. I talk to lots of men your age who have very young girlfriends or mistresses, but for most of them, the relationship is predicated on how much money and "security" the man can offer the younger woman. Clearly that's not the case for you.

The real issue here may be that your relationship has run its course, and now it's time for both of you to move on. Neither one of you sounds happy with your current situation, so sit down with Vicky and have a reality check conversation. If a relationship isn't working, trying to force it won't fix things.

This doesn't mean that you can't be friends or support each other anymore. In fact, you might find that your age difference will make you better friends than lovers in the long run, which can be a healthy and satisfying relationship. So you both need to take an adult step toward a life that makes both of you happy, even if this means parting ways.

EPILOGUE
NOW THAT YOU KNOW WHAT YOU'RE DOING...

Now that you've finished your sex education course and know what can go wrong and how to fix it, you can refer to this handy cheat sheet, which covers what your guy needs to know. It's perfect for his short attention span and perfect for you to catch any problems on the run and solve them quickly.

Part I

If he has any of these common sexual dysfunctions, explain to him that he needs to get help for them. Resolving them will spice up your sex life. Ask him gently:

- ☐ Are you overweight, especially with a big belly? Is your height more than double your waist size? Can you see your penis?
- ☐ Are your testicles small, like the size of small cherries?
- ☐ Are you getting less than six hours of sleep every night?
- ☐ Are you drinking too much alcohol, more than two drinks per day?
- ☐ Are you feeling depressed or unusually stressed?
- ☐ Do you have trouble with regular erections, especially getting or maintaining them?
- ☐ Are you ejaculating too quickly?

☐ Or are you having problems ejaculating at all? (Tell him you'll love him no matter what the answer!)

☐ Are you having sex less than your wife wants you to?

☐ Are you masturbating more than you're having sex?

☐ Would you rather watch porn than just about anything else, including spending time with your partner?

Part II

The heart of good communication and of maintaining a loving emotional relationship is with LSD = Listening + Security + Desire. If you can nail that, you can nail a fantastic sex life.

☐ Are you a good listener? If not, listen to your partner and shut the fuck up. Let her finish talking and then look her in the eyes and acknowledge that you've heard what she said.

☐ Don't fix anything she doesn't tell you she wants fixed.

☐ Make sure you provide for your partner financially. This doesn't mean you need to make a lot of money. It means that she has the confidence she needs that you will be able to provide for her in every possible way.

☐ Show her how much you desire her.

☐ Always make her feel that your relationship is more about her than about you.

When you do that, I guarantee you'll be happy, in bed and out. And so will she. Good luck to you both and, most importantly, have fun.

REFERENCES

Abt Associates Inc. "Final Report on the Evaluation of the First Offender Prostitution Program." Prepared for Karen Bachar, Office of Research and Evaluation, National Institute of Justice, March 7, 2008.

American Psychiatric Association. *Diagnostic and Statistical Manual of Mental Disorders*, 4th ed., text revision. Washington, DC: American Psychiatric Association, 2000.

"Americans Can't Put Down Their Smartphones, Even During Sex." Source: www.jumio.com/2013/07/americans-cant-put-down-their-smartphones-even-during-sex.

Atmaca M, Kuloglu M, Tezcan E, Semercioz A. "The Efficacy of Citalopram in the Treatment of Premature Ejaculation: A Placebo-Controlled Study." *International Journal of Impotence Research* 2002 Dec; 14(6):502–505.

Atwood JD, Schwartz L. "Cyber-Sex: The New Affair; Treatment Considerations." *Journal of Couple and Relationship Therapy.* 2002; 1(3):37–56.

Awwad Z, Abu-Hijleh M, Basri S, Shegam N, Murshidi M, Ajlouni K. "Penile Measurements in Normal Adult Jordanians and in Patients with Erectile Dysfunction." *Int J Impot Res* 2005 Mar-Apr; 17(2):191–195.

Berger GS, Goldstein M, Fuerst M. *The Couple's Guide to Fertility*, 3rd ed. New York: Broadway Books, 2001.

Berman JR, Berman LA, Toler SM, Gill J, Haughie S; Sildenafil Study Group. "Safety and Efficacy of Sildenafil Citrate for the Treatment of Female Sexual Arousal Disorder: A Double-Blind, Placebo Controlled Study." *Journal of Urology* 2003 Dec; 170(6, Pt 1):2333–2338.

Bhasin S, Buckwalter JG. "Testosterone Supplementation in Older Men: A Rational Idea Whose Time Has Not Yet Come." *Journal of Andrology* 2001; 22:718–731.

Brambilla DJ, O'Donnell AB, Matsumoto AM, McKinlay JM. "Lack of Seasonal Variation in Serum Sex Hormone Levels in Middle-Aged to Older Men in the Boston Area." *Journal of Clinical Endocrinology & Metabolism* 2007; 92(11):4224–4229.

"The Business of Smut: What Is It Worth?" Sources: Adams Media Research, Forrester Research, Veronis Suhler Communications Industry Report, IVD.

Buswell L, Zabriskie R, Lundberg N, Hawkins A. "The Relationship Between Father Involvement in Family Leisure and Family Functioning: The Importance of Daily Family Leisure." *Leisure Sciences: An Interdisciplinary Journal.* 2012; 34(2): pp. 172–190.

Carvalho J, Quinta-Gomes A, Laja P, Oliveira C, Vilarinho S, Janssen E, & Nobre, P. (In press). "Gender Differences in Sexual Arousal and Emotional Responses to Erotica: The Effect of Type of Film and Instructions." *Archives of Sexual Behavior.*

Center for Sexual Health Promotion, Indiana University. "Findings from the National Survey of Sexual Health and Behavior (NSSHB)." *Journal of Sexual Medicine* 2010 Oct; 7 (Suppl 5):243–373.

Chang J. *The Tao of Love and Sex.* New York: E. P. Dutton, 1977, p. 21.

Cohen A, Wong ML, Resnick D. "Localized Seminal Plasma Protein Hypersensitivity." *Allergy and Asthma Proceedings* 2004 Jul-Aug; 25(4):261–262.

Cooper A, Scherer C, Boies S, Gordon B. *Sexuality on the Internet: From Sexual Exploration to Pathological Expression.* 1999; 30(2):154–164.

Dabbs JM, LaRue D, Williams PM. "Testosterone and Occupational Choice: Actors, Ministers, and Other Men." *Journal of Personality and Social Psychology* 1990; 59:1261–1265.

Demark-Wahnefried W, et al. "Serum Androgens: Associations with Prostate Cancer Risk and Hair Patterning." *J Androl* 1998 Sep-Oct; 19(5):631.

Diamond J. "Everything Else You Ever Wanted to Know about Sex." *Discover Magazine*, April 1985, p. 73, column 1.

Edwards S, Carne C. "Oral Sex and Transmission of Non-Viral STIs. *Sexually Transmitted Infections* 1998; 74(2):95–100.

Endogenous Hormones and Prostate Cancer Collaborative Group. "Endogenous Sex Hormones and Prostate Cancer: A Collaborative Analysis of 18 Prospective Studies." *Journal of the National Cancer Institute* 2008; 100:170–183.

Eskenazi B, Wyrobek AJ, Sloter E, Kidd SA, Moore L, Young S. "The Association of Age and Semen Quality in Healthy Men." *Human Reproduction* 2003; 18(2):447–454.

Feldman HA, Goldstein I, Hatzichristou DG, Krane RJ, McKinlay JB. "Impotence and Its Medical and Psychosocial Correlates: Results of the Massachusetts Male Aging Study." *J Urol* 1994; 151:54–61.

Fisch H, Braun S. *The Male Biological Clock*. New York: The Free Press, 2005, p. 3.

Fisch H, Hyun G, Hensle TW. "Testicular Growth and Gonadotrophin Response Associated with Varicocele Repair in Adolescent Males." *BJU International* 2003 January; 91(1):75–78.

Gorelick JI, Goldstein M. "Loss of Fertility in Men with Varicocele." *Fertility and Sterility* 1993; 59(3):613–616.

Griffin G. *Penis Size and Enlargement: Facts, Fallacies, and Proven Methods.* Aptos, CA: Hourglass, 1995.

Halvorsen BL, Holte K, Myhrstad MC, et al. "A Systematic Screening of Total Antioxidants in Dietary Plants." *Journal of Nutrition* 2002; 132:461–471.

Hamilton, T. *Skin Flutes and Velvet Gloves*. New York: St. Martin's Press, 2002.

Handelsman DJ, Conway AJ, Radonic I, Turtle JR. "Prevalence, Testicular Function and Seminal Parameters in Men with Sperm Antibodies." *Clinical Reproduction and Fertility* 1983; 2(1):39–45.

Herman LM, Miner MM, Quallich SA. "Testosterone Deficiency in Men: Update on Treatment Strategies." *Practicing Clinicians Exchange* 2010; 1(2):1–8.

Houston, Ruth. *Is He Cheating on You? 829 Telltale Signs*. New York, NY: Lifestyle Publications, 2002.

Jackson AL, Murphy LL. "Role of the Hypothalamic-Pituitary-Adrenal Axis in the Suppression of Luteinizing Hormone Release by Delta-9-Tetrahydrocannabinol." *Neuroendocrinology* 1997; 65:446–452.

Janssen, E. (2011). "Sexual arousal in men: A review and conceptual analysis." *Hormones and Behavior*, doi:10.1016/j.yhbeh.2011.03.004.

Jiang M, Xin J, Zou Q, Shen JW. "A Research on the Relationship between Ejaculation and Serum Testosterone Level in Men." *Journal of Zhejiang University. Science* 2003; 4(2):236–240.

Patrick DL, et al. "Premature Ejaculation: An Observational Study of Men and Their Partners." *J Sex Med* 2005; 2:358–367.

Jones JC, Barlow DH. "Self-Reported Frequency of Sexual Urges, Fantasies, and Masturbatory Fantasies in Heterosexual Males and Females." *Arch Sex Behav* 1990 Jun; 19(3):269–79.

Joy JE, Watson SJ, Benson JA, eds. *Marijuana and Medicine: Assessing the Science Base.* Washington, DC: National Academy Press, 1999, p. 104.

Karabinus DS. "Chromatin Structural Changes in Sperm after Scrotal Insulation of Holstein Bulls." *J Androl* 1997 Sep-Oct; 18(5):549–555.

Kidd SA, Eskenazi B, Wyrobek AJ. "Effects of Male Age on Semen Quality and Fertility: A Review of the Literature." *Fertility and Sterility* 2001; 75(2):237–248.

Kinsey AC, Pomeroy WB, Martin CE. *Sexual Behavior in the Human Male.* Philadelphia: WB Saunders Co., 1948.

Koutsky L. "Epidemiology of Genital Human Papillomavirus Infection. "*American Journal of Medicine* 1997, 102(5A), 3–8.

Laumann E, Gagnon JH, Michael RT, Michaels S. *The Social Organization of Sexuality: Sexual Practices in the United States.* Chicago: University of Chicago Press, 1994.

Layden MA. (Center for Cognitive Therapy, Department of Psychiatry, University of Pennsylvania), Testimony for U.S. Senate Committee on Commerce, Science and Transportation, November 18, 2004, 2.

Levin RJ. "The Physiology of Sexual Arousal in the Human

Female: A Recreational and Procreational Synthesis." *Arch Sex Behav* 2002 Oct; 31(5):405–11.

Marieb EN. *Human Anatomy and Physiology*, 2nd ed. Redwood City, CA: Benjamin Cummings Publishing Co., 1992, p. 501.

Maslow, AH. "A Theory of Human Motivation." *Psychological Review*, Vol 50(4), Jul 1943, 370–396.

Masters WH, Johnson VE. *Human Sexual Response.* Boston: Little, Brown & Co., 1966.

Mayo Clinic Health Information website. Available at: www.mayoclinic.com/health/hydrocele/DS00617/DSECTION=7 Accessed 9/17/09.

Ménézo YJ, Hazout A, Panteix G, et al. "Antioxidants to Reduce Sperm DNA Fragmentation: An Unexpected Adverse Effect." *Reproductive Biomedicine Online* 2007;14(4):418–421.

NOW Toronto magazine. *Love and Sex Guide and Survey*, 2004.

Orakwe JC, Ogbuagu BO, Ebuh GU. "Can Physique and Gluteal Size Predict Penile Length in Adult Nigerian Men?" *West African Journal of Medicine* 2006 Jul-Sep; 25(3):223–225.

Owusu-Edusei K, et al. "The Estimated Direct Medical Cost of Selected Sexually Transmitted Infections in the United States, 2008." *Sex Transm Dis* 2013; 40(3):197–201.

Pinkerton SD, Bogart LM, Cecil H, Abramson PR. (2002). "Factors Associated with Masturbation in a Collegiate Sample." *Journal of Psychology and Human Sexuality* 2002; 14(2/3):103–121.

Reichenberg A, et al. "Advancing Paternal Age and Autism." *Archives of General Psychiatry* 2006; 63:1026–1032.

Rhoden EL, Morgentaler A. "Risks of Testosterone-Replacement Therapy and Recommendations for Monitoring." *New England Journal of Medicine* 2004; 350:482–492.

Robbins C, Schick V, Reece M, Herbenick D, Sanders, S, Dodge, B, & Fortenberry, JD. (in press). "Prevalence, Frequency, and Associations of Masturbation with Other Sexual Behaviors among Adolescents Living in the United States of America." *Archives of Pediatric and Adolescent Medicine.*

Saltzman EA, Guay AT, Jacobson J. "Improvement in Erectile Function in Men with Organic Erectile Dysfunction by Correction of Elevated Cholesterol Levels: A Clinical Observation." *J Urol* 2004 July; 172(1):255–258.

Satterwhite CL, et al. "Sexually Transmitted Infections among U.S. Women and Men: Prevalence and Incidence Estimates, 2008." *Sex Transm Dis* 2013; 40(3):187–193.

Schover LR, Thomas AJ, Jr. *Overcoming Male Infertility: Understanding its Causes and Treatments.* New York: John Wiley & Sons, 2000, p. 36.

Seidel HM, Ball JW, Dains JE, Benedict GW. *Mosby's Guide to Physical Examination*, 4th ed. St. Louis: Mosby Inc., 1999.

Shabsigh R, Rowland D. The *Diagnostic and Statistical Manual of Mental Disorders*, Fourth Edition, Text Revision as an Appropriate Diagnostic for Premature Ejaculation. *J Sex Med* 2007; 4:1468–1478.

Shamloul R. "Treatment of Men Complaining of Short Penis." *Urology* 2005; 65(6):1183–1185.

Sharlip D. "New Therapies for Erectile Dysfunction. Medscape Urology," at www.medscape.com/viewarticle/459656 Accessed February 2, 2004.

Smith TW. American Sexual Behavior: Trends, Socio-Demographic Differences, and Risk Behavior. National Opinion Research Center, University of Chicago. GSS Topical Report No. 25. Updated March 2006.

Sokhi DS, Hunter MD, Wilkinson ID, Woodruff, PWR. "Male and Female Voices Activate Distinct Regions in the Male Brain." NeuroImage 27 (2005): 572–578.

Stack S, Wasserman I, Kern R. "Adult Social Bonds and Use of Internet Pornography." *Social Science Quarterly* 2004; 85:75–88.

Stulhofer A. "How (Un)Important Is Penis Size for Women with Heterosexual Experience?" *Arch Sex Behav* 2006; 35(1):5.

Tang WS, Khoo EM. "Prevalence and Correlates of Premature Ejaculation in a Primary Care Setting: A Preliminary Cross-Sectional Study." *J Sex Med* 2011; 7:2017–2018.

Thayer RE. *The Origin of Everyday Moods.* New York: Oxford University Press USA, 1996.

Tsai EC, Matsumoto AM, Fujimoto WY, Boyko EJ. "Association of Bioavailable, Free, and Total Testosterone with Insulin Resistance." *Diabetes Care* 2004; 27:861–868.

University of California at Santa Barbara SexInfo site. www.soc.ucsb.edu/sexinfo/?article=hKjl Accessed 8/21/07.

Vale J. "Benign Prostatic Hyperplasia and Erectile Dysfunction—Is There a Link?" *Current Medical Research and Opinion* 2000; 16(Suppl 1):s63–s67.

Weinstock H, Berman S, Cates W Jr. "Sexually Transmitted Diseases among American Youth: Incidence and Prevalence Estimates, 2000." *Perspectives on Sexual and Reproductive Health* 2004; 36(1):6–10.

Wessells H, Lue TF, McAninch JW. "Penile Length in the Flaccid and Erect States: Guidelines for Penile Augmentation." *J Urol* 1996 Sep; 156(3):995–997.

Wilson GT, Lawson DM. "Expectancies, Alcohol, and Sexual Arousal in Male Social Drinkers." *Journal of Abnormal Psychology* 1976; 85:587–594.

Young S. "The Subtle Side of Sex." *New Scientist,* August 14, 1993, 24–27.

INDEX

A

abdominal fat, 65, 93–97, 102–103, 125, 127–128

acne, 71

addiction
food, 66–68
online fantasy gaming, 247–248
sex, 137, 162–165
social media, 157–159
Viagra, 115–116
See also porn

affairs. See cheating

aggression. See control in relationship

aging, 69, 106–116
"angle of the dangle," 45, 108
average frequency of sex, 10–11
erectile dysfunction, 41, 45, 89–90, 107–108, 110
erection-enhancing drugs (EEDs), 45, 109–116
sex drive, 89–90, 106–109
sleep apnea, 124
testosterone levels, 45, 89–90, 107–108, 110
women, 34, 85, 107, 108

alcohol, 29, 40, 87, 90, 119–120, 122, 124, 187

alkyl nitrites, 121

American Sexual Behavior Study, 8, 10–11

American Sexual Health Association, 160

anabolic steroids, 118

anatomy, 77–79

anger, 216

"angle of the dangle," 45, 108

antidepressants, 27, 29, 34, 118

antioxidants, 98

anxiety, performance, 39–47, 110, 207–208

aphrodisiacs, 120–122

Astroglide, 35

atrophic vaginitis, 85–86

average daily erections, 8

average frequency of masturbation, 21

average frequency of sex, 8–11

average length of sex act, 9–10

average penis size, 81

average testicle size, 128

B

baldness, 220–221

Bartoli, Marion, 94

benzocaine, 32

bioflavonoids, 98

biological clock, female, 179–182

biological versus chronological clock, 107–109

bipolar disorder, 57

birth control, 131–132, 201
   See also condoms

blood tests, basic, 117–118

body hair, removal of, 63–64, 68–69

body image, 28–29, 135, 216

body language, 178, 185–186, 236–237

body type related to penis size, 82

Botox injections, 69

brain processes, 177, 182–183

Brando, Marlon, 35

Brazilians, 63

breast implants, 135, 235–236

breathing techniques, 184

buried penis syndrome, 102–103

C

calorie intake, 103–104

cardiovascular health, 78–79

caring, xv–xvi, 219

cell phones, prepaid, 154

cell phones, turning off, 73, 74–76

CEOs, 210–211

cheating
   breast implants, 235–236
   cybersex, 155–157
   emotional cheating, 146–147, 155–159
   fantasies during masturbation, 25–26, 156
   fantasy role-play, 245–246

   gay men still in the closet, 62
   jumping to conclusions, 51
   performance anxiety, 46
   porn as, 146–147
   prostitutes, 23–24, 51, 163–164
   quiz, 152–153
   reasons for, 154–155
   sex addiction, 137, 163
   sexual frustration, 228–230
   sexually transmitted infections, 159–160
   social media, 157–159
   statistics on, 154
   strip clubs, 161–162, 163–164

cheat sheets, 259–260

checklist, sex, 17

chlamydia, 160

chronic masturbation, 17–23
   as cheating, 25–26
   dealing with, 27, 38, 143, 147–148, 149, 227–228
   inability to orgasm with partner, 20, 21–23, 37–38, 135, 141–143, 226–228
   porn, 135, 136–137, 141–143, 147–148
   premature ejaculation, 20, 22, 27
   psychology and physiology, 20–23
   retarded ejaculation, 37–38, 142–143, 226–228

chronological versus biological clock, 107–109

Cialis, 111, 115–116
   See also erection-enhancing drugs (EEDs)

Claritin D, 119

cleanliness, 69–70, 189–190, 234

clitoris, 28, 30, 34, 78–79, 81

clothes, 71–72

cocaine, 120, 121–122

codeine, 118, 119

coffee, 87

communication
  aging, 108–109
  lubrication, need for, 35–36
  performance anxiety, 42–43
  sex positions, 6–8
  stress, 53
  See also LSD (listening+security+desire)
compliments, 14–15, 192–193, 197
compromising, 169, 200–202, 229, 240–242, 246, 255
compulsive behaviors, 162–163
concealer, 71
condoms, 35, 41, 130, 131, 160, 201–202
confidence. See performance anxiety
congenital conditions, 89
continuous positive airway pressure (CPAP), 124–125
control in relationship, 42–43, 207–209, 226–228, 249–250
cooling down, 187, 191
Cosmopolitan magazine, 13
counselors, marital, 62, 140, 187, 191
CPAP (continuous positive airway pressure), 124–125
cramps, 28, 50
cybersex, 155–157, 163

D

dandruff, 70
dark under-eye circles, 71
date nights, 230–232, 255–256
deep breathing, 184
delicate topics, bringing up, 195–198
denial, 3 4, 24, 137, 140, 145, 229

deodorant, 69
depression, 51, 53, 56–58, 92, 99, 256–258
desire, 233–258
  breast implants, 235–236
  catching your patterns, 251–256
  dominatrixes, 256–258
  expressing, 236–240
  Five Things I Desire list, 238–239
  "How Much Desire Each Other" scale, 236–237
  overview, xvii, 168–169, 233–234
  spicing up your sex life, 46–47, 134, 240–248, 253–256
  submission/dominance, 243–244, 249–250
  thoughtfulness and caring, 13–15
  See also sex drive; sex turn offs
diet
  fatigue, cause of, 89
  food addiction, 66–68
  foods for sexual prowess, 98
  for health weight and muscle gain, 100–102, 104
  men versus women, 103–104
  semen, taste of, 87
  testosterone levels, 90, 93–94, 103
  for weight loss, 18–19, 68, 95, 96–97, 100
  weight-loss plateau, 99–100
digital devices
  cheating, 154
  turning off, 73, 74–76, 247–248
dildos, 247
dipstick, sex as, vii–viii, xii–xiv
diseases, 117–119, 159–160
dismissive attitude, 178, 180–181, 202–203, 219, 221
divorce, 40–42

doctor-shopping, 112

Dole, Bob, 109

dominant role-play, 243–244

dominatrixes, 256–258

Dr. Oz Show, The, xi

drugs, medical. See medication; OTC (over-the-counter) drugs

drugs, recreational, 40, 87, 90, 119–122, 256–258

dryness. See lubrication

E

ego-driven versus ego-appropriate attitude, 219

ejaculation. See erectile dysfunction; masturbation; orgasms; premature ejaculation; semen

electronic devices
cheating, 154
turning off, 73, 74–76, 247–248

emasculation. See control in relationship

embracing attitude, 219

emotional cheating, 146–147, 155–159

emotional impediments, 146, 156–157

emotional intelligence, 176–177

emotional relationship, viii–xii
See also LSD (listening+security+desire)

emotional security. See security

energy supplements, 27–28

equipment compatibility, 85–86

erectile dysfunction
aging, 41, 45, 89–90, 107–108, 110
medications, caused by, 118–119
performance anxiety, 39–47, 110, 207–208

recreational drugs and alcohol, 40, 90, 119–122

statistics on, 110

younger men, 41, 42–43

See also erection-enhancing drugs (EEDs); testosterone

erection-enhancing drugs (EEDs)
aging, 45, 109–116
buying on Internet, 114–115
dosage/effects, 111, 115–116
low testosterone and, 110, 111, 113
mechanism of action, 110–111
overuse, 111–116
penis width, 84–85
for performance anxiety, 42, 43, 45, 110, 207–208
See also Viagra

erections
"angle of the dangle," 45, 108
average daily number of, 8
"breaking" your penis, 80
foods for sexual prowess, 98
medication, inhibited by, 118–119
in morning, 41–42, 79–80, 106
penis health, needed for, 78, 141
physiology of, 77–79
semen, 86–87
size of penis, 80–86
during sleep, 78, 79–80
See also erectile dysfunction; sex drive; testosterone

estrogen replacement therapy, 34

exercise, 103–106
diet and, 101–102
getting motivated for, 67–68, 105–106
raising testosterone levels, 89, 90, 96, 101, 102, 103, 104
sleep needs, 102
stress-busting, 222

weight training, 102, 104–105
women, 104, 229
exercises, Kegel, 32–33
ex-girlfriends/wives, 202–203
exhaustion, 50, 89–90, 91, 122–126
eye bags, 71

F

Facebook, 157–159
fake relationships, 207–208
faking orgasms, 39
fantasizing during masturbation, 25–26, 156
fantasy role-play, 241–248
fatigue, 50, 89–90, 91, 122–126
feminine hygiene products, 29
Fifty Shades of Grey (James), 243–244
financial security, xvi–xvii, 168, 205–211, 212, 222–226
fish, 102
five-point checkup, 117–118
five rules for sexual security, 214–216
"five things" lists
    desires, 238–239
    sex needs/wants, 204
"fix-it" mentality, 177, 184, 185, 188
food. See diet
foreplay
    communication, 189
    condoms, 35
    encouraging personal grooming, 68–69, 70, 72, 190
    lubrication, 86
    masturbation, 31, 38, 143
    thoughtfulness and caring, 13–15, 252–253
frequency of sex, xii–xiv, 8–11, 106

G

games, online fantasy, 247–248
gay men still in the closet, 59–65
generosity, 213–214
gift of thoughtfulness, 216–218
giving back, 213–214
Godfather, The, 85–86
good sex, as skill, 4–8, 16–17
grooming, 63–64, 68–72, 189–190, 234
grudges, 216

H

hair care, 70
happiness, ix
HEAD acronym, 87–88
herpes, 160
hobbies, 222
homosexuals still in the closet, 59–65
hormones. See menopause; testosterone; testosterone replacement therapy
household chores, 13–14, 213–214, 252–253
Houston, Ruth, 154
Howard 101 channel, xi
"How Much Desire Each Other" scale, 236–237
HPV (human papilloma virus), 160
humanism, 14–15
human papilloma virus (HPV), 160
hygiene and grooming, 63–64, 68–72, 189–190, 234
hypogonadism, 89–90
    See also testosterone

I

idiosyncratic masturbation, 37–38
immaturity, 199–200, 251–253
infertility, 93, 126–128, 179–182
Internet
  buying prescription drugs on, 114–115
  misinformation about sex, 11, 12
  porn, 11, 133, 135–136, 155–157
Is He Cheating on You? 829 Telltale Signs
  (Houston), 154
"I" versus "you" statements, 186

J

job-related stress, 43–45, 53–55
judgmental attitude, 214, 219, 245
juvenile attitude, 199–200

K

kefir, 101–102
Kegel exercises, 32–33
Kinsey, Alfred, 9
Kinsey Institute, 21
Klondike ads, 182
K-Y Jelly, 35

L

Last Tango in Paris, 35
latex condoms, 35
Leary, Timothy, 167
LeBron, James, 102
length, penis, 80–86
length of sex act, average, 9–10
Levitra, 111, 115–116
  See also erection-enhancing drugs (EEDs)

libido. See desire; sex drive; sex turn
  offs; testosterone
lidocaine spray, 32
listening, 171–204
  backing off and cooling down, 187, 191
  bad communication patterns, 198–203
  body language, 178, 185–186, 236–237
  communication strategies for women,
    193–198
  compliments, 14–15, 192–193, 197
  compromising, 169, 200–202, 229, 240–242,
    246, 255
  delicate topics, bringing up, 195–198
  "five things I need during sex" list, 204
  male brain processes, 177, 182–183
  men talking with other men, 191–192
  men versus women, 176–177
  overview, xvi, 168
  poker, compared to, 185–186
  rules for guys, 183–185, 186–188
  shut the f*** up, 171–182
lists
  fantasies, 245
  Five Things I Desire, 238–239
  I Need Five Things During Sex, 204
LSD (listening+security+desire), xv–
  xviii, 5, 167–169, 260
  See also desire; listening; security
lubrication
  for controlling premature ejaculation, 27, 36
  types, 35
  vaginal, 33–36, 85–86, 108

M

male biological clock, 107–109
man boobs, 66
manners, 72–73, 217

marijuana, 87, 120, 122

marital counselors, 62, 140, 187, 191

married couples, frequency of sex for, 8–9, 10

Maslow's Pyramid of Needs, 212–214

Masters and Johnson, 82

masturbation
average frequency of, 21
as cheating, 25–26, 156
psychology and physiology, 20–23
sex addiction, 162
women, 21, 28–31
See also chronic masturbation

media, 28–29, 109

medical tests, basic, 117–118

medication
for baldness, 220–221
for controlling premature ejaculation, 27–28, 32, 36
for excessive sweating, 69
Internet, buying on, 114–115
media, 28–29
sexual health, negative effect on, 89, 118–119
testosterone replacement therapy, 18, 90–93, 99, 111, 122, 127, 128
vaginal dryness, 34
See also erection-enhancing drugs (EEDs)

menopause, 34, 46–47, 85, 107, 108, 228–230

menstruation, 28–29, 50

metabolism, 104, 105, 126

methamphetamines, 121–122

military, 210, 224–226

money. See financial security

morning erections, 41–42, 79–80, 106

Motivation and Personality (Maslow), 212

myths, 30, 82

N

narcissism, 73, 137, 154, 164

National Sleep Foundation (NSF), 122

natural lubricants, 35

nest-building, 222–224

Nicholson, Harold, 216

nighttime urination, 123

nitric oxide, 78, 98, 110

nocturnal penile tumescence, 79–80

non-prescription drugs. See OTC (over-the-counter) drugs

O

obesity, 18–19, 65–68, 74, 102–103, 127–128, 234

oil-based lubricants, 35

omega-3 fatty acids, 102

opiates, 120, 122

oral sex, 86–87, 246

orgasms
average length of sex act, 9–10
clitoral lubrication, 34
lack of, by women, 5, 6
medication, inhibited by, 118–119
physiology of, 77–79
retarded ejaculation, 19–20, 37–38, 142–143, 226–228
semen, 86–87
sex positions, 6–8
vaginal penetration and, 6, 9, 30, 81, 82–84
See also premature ejaculation

OTC (over the-counter) drugs
   aphrodisiacs, 120–122
   premature ejaculation, controlling, 27–28, 32, 36
   sexual health, negative effect on, 119

P

painkillers, 118, 119, 122

pedometers, 67–68, 105

pencil dicks, 85

penis
   body type, related to, 82
   "breaking," 80
   equipment compatibility, 85–86
   physiology of, 77–79
   size, 80–86
   See also erections

performance anxiety, 39–47, 110, 207–208

perfume, 64

perimenopause, 34, 107

period, monthly, 28–29, 50

personal hygiene, 68–71, 189–190, 234

Peyronie's disease, 80

pheromones, 63–64

pill popping, 111–114

pituitary tumors, 91, 126

pleasing your partner first, 215, 246

poker game, 185–186

politeness, 72–73, 217

"poppers," 121

porn, 132–152
   chronic masturbation, 135, 136–137, 141–143, 147–148, 149
   cybersex, 155–157, 163
   dealing with addiction, 142–143, 144–146, 147–152
   effect on sexual performance, 140–141
   emotional cheating, 146–147
   versus emotional connection, 135, 136–137, 146–147, 149
   Internet, 11, 133, 135–136, 155–157
   in moderation, 134, 242–243
   proliferation of, 132–133
   psychological effects, 135–137, 143–144
   quiz, 138–139
   retarded ejaculation, 19–20, 142–143
   sex addiction, 163
   unrealistic expectations, 11, 12, 19–20, 135–136, 143–144, 241

positions, sex, 6–8, 27

positive attitude/energy, 195, 197, 217

practicing good sex, 16–17

PreBoost Lubricating Warming Gel, 36

pregnancy, 254
   infertility, 93, 126–128, 179–182
   lubricants, inhibited by, 34–35
   penis size, 83

premature ejaculation
   chronic masturbation, 20, 22, 27
   controlling, 27–28, 32–33, 36
   definition, 26–27
   denial, 3–4, 24
   gay men still in the closet, 60–61
   prostitutes, 23–24
   statistics on, 5, 9

probiotics, 102

prolactin levels, 125–126

props, 247

prostate health, 92–93, 117, 123, 141

prostitutes, 23–24, 51, 163–164

protein, dietary, 101–102

PSA (prostate-specific antigen), 117

pseudoephedrine, 119

Q

quizzes
cheating, 152–153
depression, 56
low testosterone, 58
porn addiction, 138–139
stress, 52

R

radio show, xi, xviii, 49, 163

reflective listening, 187

relaxation techniques, 40, 184

respectfulness, 72–73, 217

retarded ejaculation, 19–20, 37–38, 142–143, 226–228

risk-taking, 129, 214–215

role-play, fantasy, 241–248

rosacea, 71

rudeness, 73

rules for listening, 183–185, 186–188

rules for sexual security, 214–216

S

safe sex habits, 41, 129–132, 160–161

salmon, 102

satisfaction, 3–47

scent, 63–64

security, 162, 205–232
attitude and, 218–219
catching your patterns, 224–230
creating your own nest, 222–224

date nights, 230–232, 255–256
Maslow's Pyramid of Needs, 212–214
need for, 206–209
overview, xvi–xvii, 168, 205–206
performance anxiety, 39–47, 110, 207–208
sexual security, rules for, 214–216
stress and, 221–222
thoughtfulness and caring, 13–15, 216–218
trust, 209–211

self-actualization, 213–214

self-image, 28–29, 216

semen, 86–87

sex, frequency of, xii–xiv, 8–11, 106

sex act, average length of, 9–10

sex addiction, 137, 162–165

sex as a skill, 4–8, 16–17

sex as dipstick of relationship, vii–viii, xii–xiv

sex checklist, 17

sex drive
abdominal fat, 65, 93–97, 102–103, 125, 127–128
aging, 89–90, 106–109
depression, 51, 53, 56–58, 92, 256–258
diseases, 117 118
erections, anatomy of, 77–79
fluctuations in, 49–50
food for sexual prowess, 98
frequency of sex, xii–xiv, 8–11, 106
HEAD acronym, 87–88
infertility, 93, 126–128, 179–182
medications, negative effects of, 89, 118–119
morning erections, 41–42, 79–80, 106
recreational drugs and alcohol, 40, 90, 119–122
sleep deprivation, 74, 102, 122–126
testosterone, related to, 88–89
weight loss, 18–19, 93–100, 102–103, 124, 125

women, xiii–xiv, 5–6

See also desire; diet; exercise; sex turn offs; testosterone

sex education, viii–xi, 11–13, 28, 77–79

sex life, spicing up, 46–47, 134, 240–248, 253–256

sex positions, 6–8, 27

sexting, 137

sex toys, 30–31, 247

sex turn offs, 49–76

digital devices, addiction to, 74–76, 247–248

exhaustion, 50, 89–90, 91, 122–126

gay men still in the closet, 59–65

manners, 72–73, 217

obesity/weight problems, 65–68, 127–128, 234

overview, 49–50

personal hygiene and grooming, 68–72, 189–190, 234

primary causes of, 49–51

quizzes, 52, 56, 58–59, 138–139, 152–153

snoring, 73–74

stress, 40–45, 52–55, 221–222

unsatisfying sex, xiii–xiv, 5–6

See also cheating; porn; sex drive; testosterone

sexual dependency, 162–163

sexual dysfunction. See chronic masturbation; erectile dysfunction; erection-enhancing drugs (EEDs); porn; premature ejaculation; sex drive; sex turn offs; testosterone; vaginal lubrication

sexual equipment compatibility, 85–86

sexually transmitted infections (STIs), 159–160

shaving, 63–64, 68–69

silent treatment, 181

Size Matters: The Hard Facts about Male Sexuality That Every Woman Should Know (Fisch), 80–81

skin cancer, 70

skin care, 70–71

sleep, erections during, 78, 79–80

sleep, for weight gain, 102

sleep apnea, 74, 123–126

sleep deprivation, 74, 102, 122–126

smart sex habits, 41, 129–132, 160–161

smell. See personal hygiene

smoking, 40, 87, 90, 120, 124

snoring, 73–74

soap, deodorant, 69–70

social media, 157–159

solutions, focusing on, 196, 201

Spanish fly, 121

sperm, 86–87, 108, 127, 128

spicing up your sex life, 46–47, 134, 240–248, 253–256

Stern, Howard, xi

steroids, 118

STIs (sexually transmitted infections), 159–160

stop-and-start technique, 27

stress, 40–45, 52–55, 187, 196, 221–222, 236–237

stress-busters, 222

strip clubs, 161–162, 163–164

submission/dominance, 243–244, 249–250

Sudafed, 119

sugars and starches, 18–19, 95, 96–97, 100

sunscreen, 70

supportive attitude, 219

surgery to increase penis length, 84

sweating, excessive, 69–70

T

testicles, size of, 128

testicles, undescended, 89

testosterone

   abdominal fat, 65, 93–97, 125, 127–128

   aging, 45, 89–90, 107–108, 110

   congenital conditions, 89

   depression, related to, 92, 99

   diet and, 90, 93–94, 103

   erection-enhancing drugs, 110, 111, 113

   exercise, 89, 90, 96, 101, 102, 103, 104

   infertility, 93, 127–128

   low, symptoms of, 58, 89–90, 94, 99, 128

   medications, negative effects of, 89, 118–119

   morning erections, 79–80

   normal ranges, 88

   personality, influence on, 89, 92–93

   quiz, 58

   sex drive, related to, 88–89

   side effects, 92–93, 122, 127, 128

   sleep deprivation, 74, 102, 123–126

   testing for, 88, 89

   See also erectile dysfunction; testosterone replacement therapy

testosterone replacement therapy, 90–93, 111

   methods of delivery, 91

   misconceptions about, 18

   side effects, 92–93, 122, 127, 128

weight loss, 99

text messages

   cheating, 157–159

   foreplay, 74

   sex addiction, 137

   turning off digital devices, 73, 74–76

therapists, 62, 140, 187, 191

thirty-year itch, 228–230

thoughtfulness, 13–15, 216–218

threesomes, 60–61, 135, 245–246

thyroid function, 125–126

tiredness, 50, 89–90, 91, 122–126

trust, 209–211

turn offs. See sex turn offs

U

undescended testicles, 89

unsatisfying sex, xiii–xiv, 5–6

urinary flow medications, 118

urinary tract infections, 87

urination, nighttime, 123

U.S. Food and Drug Administration, 32, 91

V

vacations, 230–231

vacuum devices, 84

vagina, size of, 81, 85–86

vaginal lubrication, 33–36, 85–86, 108

vaginal penetration, and orgasms, 6, 9, 30, 81, 82–84

vaginoplasty, 86

varicocele, 89

vegan diet, 100

Viagra, 23–24

aging, 45, 109–116
dosage/effects, 111, 115–116
penis width, 84–85
performance anxiety, 42, 43, 45, 110, 207–208
as quick fix, ix–x, 5
See also erection-enhancing drugs (EEDs)
vibrators, 30–31, 247
vitamins, 27–28, 96
"Vitamin V." See erection-enhancing drugs (EEDs)

W
waist size, ideal, 94
WebMD, 57
websites, xi, 57, 154
"weekender, the," 111
weight loss, 18–19, 65–68, 93–100, 102–103, 124, 125
weight-loss plateau, 99–100
weight problems
    abdominal fat, 65, 93–97, 102–103, 125, 127–128
    buried penis syndrome, 102–103
    male biological clock, 107–108
    sexual turn offs, 65–68, 127–128, 234
    sleep apnea, 74, 124, 125
    struggling for weight gain, 100–102, 104
    testosterone levels, 18, 66, 127–129
    See also diet; weight loss
weight training, 102, 104–105
Weiner, Anthony, 137
women
    aging, 34, 85, 107, 108
    average time to orgasm, 9–10
    body image, 28–29, 135, 216
    cheating, reasons for, 154, 155
    clitoris, anatomy of, 78–79

faking orgasms, 39
masturbation, 21, 28–31
perimenopause/menopause, 34, 46–47, 85, 107, 228–230
self-blame, 23, 24, 37, 165
sex positions, 6–8
submission fantasies, 243–244
unsatisfying sex, xiii–xiv, 5–6
vaginal lubrication, 33–36, 85–86, 108
vagina size, 81, 85–86
vibrators, 30–31, 247
weight training, 104
work-related stress, 43–45, 53–55
World of Warcraft, 248

Y
yogurt, 101–102

Z
Zoloft, 27

ACKNOWLEDGMENTS

I want to thank my wife, Karen, for the knowledge she has given me to write this book. Let me be honest. If it weren't for her, there would be no book. And thanks for being a great wife for thirty-two years and the best partner I can imagine. I love you!

I want to thank my children for being my children, even though they had no part in this book. I love them. (I know they do not want me to mention them by name, but they are David, Melissa, and Sam.)

Thank you, Karen Moline, for co-authoring this fantastic book. You are an immensely talented writer.

Nena Madona, my agent at Dupree-Miller, your guidance is priceless.

Stephanie Bowen, my editor at Sourcebooks. You knew instantaneously what this book means and how best to realize my vision. Also, many thanks to the rest of the Sourcebooks team for helping to make this happen.

Shuli Egar, Tim Sabean, and Jim McClure at *The Howard Stern Show*/Sirius Radio Network. You have provided a platform for people to get information in the most fun and accessible way possible. Without you guys, there would be no *Dr. Harry Fisch Show*.

Steve Carlis and Hank Norman, who have guided my radio

talents and taught me how to think and talk in the media to reach the widest possible audience.

Lastly, thanks to my patients and listeners of the *Dr. Harry Fisch Show*. Allowing me to be a part of your lives means the world to me. It's why I became a doctor in the first place.

ABOUT THE AUTHOR

Harry Fisch MD, FACS, is a board-certified urologist at New York Presbyterian Hospital, Weill Medical College of Cornell University, where he is a clinical professor of urology and reproductive medicine. He is one of the nation's leading doctors in the diagnosis and treatment of men's health issues, such as low testosterone, as well as sexuality and fertility

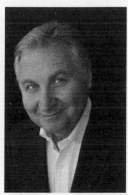
Deborah Feingold

problems. Internationally renowned, he has pioneered microsurgical techniques for disorders associated with male infertility. He has also been named to the "Best Doctors in America" and "New York Magazine Top Doctor" lists for the past nine years.

In his private practice in Manhattan, Dr. Fisch has successfully treated thousands of men and couples with sexuality and fertility problems. His research on sperm counts and endocrine disrupters has resulted in multiple research articles and international attention, and his work has frequently been cited in publications including *USA Today,* the *New York Times,* and the *Washington Post.* He has appeared on television's *60 Minutes, 20/20,* CNN, and the *Today* show, and is a regular blogger and guest on *The Dr. Oz Show* as a medical expert on men's health. Dr. Fisch is also the author of two books, *The Male Biological Clock* and *Size Matters*, and the host of the *Dr. Harry Fisch Show* on SiriusXM radio.

Karen Moline has collaborated on more than two dozen non-fiction books and is co-author of the *New York Times* bestseller, *Sh*tty Mom: The Parenting Guide for the Rest of Us*. She has also written two novels, *Lunch* and *Belladonna*, as well as hundreds of articles for publications around the globe. Her work can be found at www.karenmoline.com.